AFTA SpringerBriefs in Family Therapy

Series Editor
Carmen Knudson-Martin
Education & Counseling, Rogers Hall
Lewis & Clark Grad School
Portland, OR, USA

SpringerBriefs present concise summaries of cutting-edge research and practical applications. Featuring compact volumes of 50 to 125 pages, the series covers a range of content from professional to academic. Typical topics might include: A timely report of state-of-the art analytical techniques A bridge between new research results, as published in journal articles, and a contextual literature review A snapshot of a hot or emerging topic An in-depth case study or clinical example A presentation of core concepts that students must understand in order to make independent contributions

Tatiana Glebova • Carmen Knudson-Martin
Editors

Sociocultural Trauma and Well-Being in Eastern European Family Therapy

AFTA
American Family Therapy Academy

Springer

Editors
Tatiana Glebova
Couple and Family Therapy Program
Alliant International University
Sacramento, CA, USA

Carmen Knudson-Martin
Emerita
Lewis & Clark College
Portland, OR, USA

ISSN 2196-5528 ISSN 2196-5536 (electronic)
AFTA SpringerBriefs in Family Therapy
ISBN 978-3-031-29994-0 ISBN 978-3-031-29995-7 (eBook)
https://doi.org/10.1007/978-3-031-29995-7

This Springer imprint is published by the registered company Springer Nature Switzerland AG
The registered company address is: Gewerbestrasse 11, 6330 Cham, Switzerland

To my family, both immediate and extended, alive and gone.

Tatiana Glebova

To all families anywhere who are touched by sociocultural trauma; may you find healing and hope.

Carmen Knudson-Martin

Series Foreword

The AFTA Springer Briefs in Family Therapy is an official publication of the American Family Therapy Academy. Each volume focuses on the practice and policy implications of innovative systemic research and theory in family therapy and allied fields. Our goal is to make information about families and systemic practices in societal contexts widely accessible in a reader friendly, conversational, and practical style. AFTA's core commitment to equality, social responsibility, and justice is represented in each volume.

That personal health and well-being must be understood in context of the larger systems with which they are embedded is core to family therapy and the mission of AFTA. Nonetheless, when clients present with symptoms such as anxiety or depression, anger, substance or domestic abuse, or child behavior or relationship problems, it can be easy to focus on the individual or family aspect of their troubles and overlook the impact of factors such as war, oppression, and political instability that affect nations and groups as a whole. *Sociocultural Trauma and Well-Being in Eastern European Family Therapy* raises readers' awareness of the insidious impact of these forces and the consequences across generations, particularly on trust and the ethical nature of relationships.

The personal and professional experience shared in this volume by authors from Hungary, Russia, Romania, Moldova, and Serbia is particularly powerful as they began writing just as Russia invaded Ukraine in February 2022. Through their insight and clinical expertise, the authors offer examples of healing and resilience with guidelines for practice. Whether from Eastern Europe, another of the many other communities that suffer sociocultural trauma, or working with people that bring these family legacies, readers will take away a valuable framework for how to approach sociocultural trauma in clinical practice and a deep appreciation for the courage and inspiration reflected in each chapter.

Carmen Knudson-Martin, Series Editor
AFTA Springer Briefs in Family Therapy
Portland, Oregon

AFTA Springer Briefs in Family Therapy

A publication of the American Family Therapy Academy

Founded in 1977, the **American Family Therapy Academy** is a non-profit organization of leading family therapy teachers, clinicians, program directors, policy-makers, researchers, and social scientists dedicated to advancing systemic thinking and practices for families in their social context.

Vision

AFTA envisions a just world by transforming social contexts that promote health, safety, and well-being of all families and communities.

Mission

AFTA's mission is developing, researching, teaching, and disseminating progressive, just family therapy and family-centered practices and policies.

Acknowledgments

Although this book was conceived a while ago, the actual work started when the COVID pandemic was still in full swing at the end of 2020; and when it appeared that the crisis was finally subsiding, Russia's war of aggression against Ukraine began in February 2022. Thus, this book on the impact of sociocultural trauma on relationships in a turbulent region has itself become a product of traumatic times, which again put relationships to a harsh stress test. I hope that this volume, imperfect as it may be, will prove timely and useful to help meet the challenge of these painful times.

Not only is this book about relationships, it was also born out of relationships. It is a result of exchange of ideas and multiple collaborations over time and various locations. Its logic, therefore, is non-linear and multifactorial, reflecting the complexity of the subject. Thinking back, life paths crossings have been amazing and miraculous—I came across so many people who influenced my perspective and contributed to this book.

Without Carmen Knudson, this volume would never have happened. I am endlessly grateful to her for all the encouragement and confidence she provided, helping me overcome my doubts and fears. Most importantly, the tremendous amount of labor she put in shaping this volume was absolutely crucial. My sincere gratitude goes to all authors of the chapters for their dedication to the topic and an extensive effort they have put into their writing.

I owe a debt of gratitude to Monica McGoldrick, Mihaela Robila, and Anna Varga who have been very helpful by sharing their professional connections which allowed me to complete the team of outstanding writers for this book.

My therapeutic approach and my way of thinking about human relationships have been fundamentally shaped by the founder of contextual family therapy Ivan Boszormenyi-Nagy's writings and lifework. As the ultimate contextual therapy expert, Catherine Ducommun-Nagy has been generous in allowing me to take advantage of her knowledge and expertise in private consultations as well as reviewing Chap. 7 for accuracy in my interpretation and application of contextual family therapy.

While I cannot possibly list everyone's name, I wish to thank everybody who came to my presentations at various conferences over the years and continents because of their interest in the topic and shared their thoughts with me. My clients' and students' reflections on their families' histories and heritage were an invaluable source of inspiration. My special thanks go to my long-term friends, Yekaterina Andrejeva-Zukova and Svetlana Lomonosova, whose support has warmed my heart for years. Although this book was years in the making, it needed a dedicated temporal space to get finished. A sabbatical provided by Alliant International University where I have been teaching since 2008 allowed me to get it done.

Finally, I would like to acknowledge my family, both immediate and extended, alive and gone. Thinking about past generations, it is only now that I begin to understand what they went through and still did their best to care about each other. Their strength is within me. My husband Kirill has been my life's co-author for decades and now became a literal co-author. My daughter Aglaya supported, lovingly challenged, and inspired me in so many ways over the years. Without them I would not be who I am.

Tatiana Glebova

When I first crossed paths with Tatiana Glebova at a professional conference, I knew I had found someone whose wisdom and spirit inspired me. That we often attended the same sessions suggested we had much to learn from each other. For several years, each time I saw her I would prompt her to submit a proposal for an AFTA SpringerBrief. We discussed several different topics. When she said she had a team of Eastern European colleagues who could write about collective trauma as a result of war and massive political and economic upheavals, I was hooked. Not only did these authors include practicing family therapists, they also included historians, sociologists, family scientists, and cultural anthropologists. This multidisciplinary, multinational perspective is unusual and so valuable. I am grateful that Tatiana convinced me to sign on as co-editor of the volume and co-author of several chapters. Working with her and her team has been one of the most positive experiences of my career. I am humbled by how much I learned. Knowing that Tatiana has family in both Russia and Ukraine and that the other authors' lives were also dramatically touched by this war, I expected they would ask for an extension. None did. Thank you all! I am deeply grateful for your willingness to share so openly and to demonstrate what it means to engage professionally from a place of heart and conviction. I am honored to contribute to this important work.

Carmen Knudson-Martin

Contents

About the Editors

Tatiana Glebova, PhD, LMFT, AAMFT Approved Supervisor, is professor of COAMFTE-accredited Couple and Family Therapy program, Alliant International University, Sacramento CA, USA. She published and presented at state, national and international conferences on many topics, including contextual family therapy and transgenerational trauma. Her clinical practice includes working with families that experienced various forms of sociocultural trauma.

Carmen Knudson-Martin, PhD, LMFT, is professor emerita of Marital, Couple, and Family Therapy, Lewis & Clark College, Portland OR, USA. She has published three other books and numerous articles and chapters on the influence of the larger sociocultural context in couple and family relationships and the political and ethical implications of therapist actions on marital equality, relational development and couple therapy. Carmen is the developer of Socio-Emotional Relationship Therapy (SERT) which addresses the micro-processes by which societal power processes play out in couple relationships. She was the 2017 recipient of the Distinguished Contribution to Family Therapy Theory and Practice award from the American Academy of Family Therapy.

Contributors

Valentina Bodrug-Lungu Moldova State University, Chisinău, Moldova

Tatiana Glebova Alliant International University, Sacramento, CA, USA

Kirill Glebov Roseville, CA, USA

Gáspár György Multicultural Association of Psychology and Psychotherapy, Bucharest, Romania

Nevena Čalovska Hercog University Singidunum, Faculty of Media and Communications, Department of Psychology, Belgrade, Serbia

Tamara Džamonja Ignjatović University of Belgrade, Faculty of Philosophy, Department of Psychology, Belgrade, Serbia

Carmen Knudson-Martin Emerita, Lewis & Clark College, Portland, OR, USA

Elena V. Miskova Center of Medical Anthropology, Institute of Ethnology and Anthropology, RAS, Moscow, Russia

Biljana Stanković University of Belgrade, Faculty of Philosophy, Department of Psychology, Belgrade, Serbia

Emőke Tarján Family Systems Therapy Institute, Budapest, Hungary

Natalia Toma Moldova State University, Chisinău, Moldova

Sergiu Toma Moldova State University, Chisinău, Moldova

Smiljka Tomanović University of Belgrade, Faculty of Philosophy, Department of Psychology, Belgrade, Serbia

University of Belgrade, Faculty of Philosophy, Department of Sociology, Belgrade, Serbia

Patrik Pál Wächter The National Archives of Hungary, Szombathely, Hungary

Orsolya Wächter-Szili Budapest, Hungary

Tamás Wittmann Family Systems Therapy Institute, Budapest, Hungary

Chapter 1
Sociocultural Trauma and Relational WellBeing in the Eastern European Context

Tatiana Glebova, Carmen Knudson-Martin, and Kirill Glebov

> *Yet the histories of families cannot be separated from the histories of nations. To divide them is part of our denial.*
>
> *—Susan Griffin (1992, as cited in McGoldrick, 2019, p. 93)*

As we write, the immediate and apparent impacts of sociocultural trauma on relationships can be clearly seen now, during the time of the war in Ukraine. While directly affecting only two countries in Eastern Europe, the war has impacted the whole world. A metaphor of earthquake seems relevant in many ways. First, with that earth-shattering experience, the closer you are to the epicenter, the worse. But people far away from the epicenter experience it as well. Second, earthquakes cause deep fissures in what was solid ground, thus breaking its continuity, and also bare the underlying geological layers from previous eras, thus making visible what was hidden from the eye. Finally, earthquakes often radically change the landscape as well as survivors' way of living in their altered environment.

I (Tatiana) have been living in the United States for more than two decades. I was born and grew up in Moscow, in the then Soviet Union, present-day Russia. Consequently, my identity was Russian; however, my father was Ukrainian. Mixed Ukrainian–Russian families are very common in both countries for reasons of shared history. Their residence, in Ukraine or Russia, was often determined by economics and job opportunities. Until high school, I spent at least 3 months a year

---

T. Glebova (✉)
Alliant International University, Sacramento, CA, USA
e-mail: tglebova@alliant.edu

C. Knudson-Martin
Emerita, Lewis & Clark College, Portland, OR, USA

K. Glebov
Roseville, CA, USA

T. Glebova, C. Knudson-Martin (eds.), *Sociocultural Trauma and Well-Being in Eastern European Family Therapy*, AFTA SpringerBriefs in Family Therapy,
https://doi.org/10.1007/978-3-031-29995-7_1

with my Ukrainian grandparents in a small village. Their primary language was Ukrainian, but they spoke Russian with me since I struggled with learning Ukrainian. When I came to the United States, it was cumbersome to explain my mixed heritage, so for the most part I would simply tell people I was Russian.

I was completely heartbroken when the war started. Even though I was far removed from its hardships and horrors, living and working in California, it still felt very personal because of my family history and continuing family ties. My aunt and her two sons with their families live in Ukraine. My aunt, my Dad's youngest sister, was born in early 1942 in the territory occupied by Nazi Germany and grew up during the time of severe fighting in that area. I remember a family story about how for years after the war she would hide under the house whenever there was a sound of an airplane. In 2022 she celebrated her 80th birthday, again hiding from the bombing, this time by the Russian army. Her 10-year-old great-granddaughter was learning fast as well—whenever she heard sounds of explosions, she would tell her family, "We need to hide." This broke the hearts of her adult family members who enjoyed her dancing practices at school before the war. But the damage to the family reached further, beyond the war's dangers and hardships—our connections with some of the extended family members who lived in Russia and supported the war were also ruptured.

Families in Ukraine experience the immediate and direct effects of war in numerous ways—death or injuries of loved ones, family separation due to women and children leaving the country and many men serving in the army, and destruction of homes and material resources, to name a few. As families and individuals live through the unthinkable, they experience shock, stress, confusion, anxiety, fear, and grief. While dealing with or putting aside their own feelings and challenges, parents try their best to protect and support their children. The elderly and those with disabilities or chronic conditions have extra challenges. If they have relatives who can help them, there are often hard dilemmas for all—staying together in a dangerous place or separating. And when relatives decide not to leave their vulnerable family members, they face hardships of finding needed medications and provisions. Some families and individuals have more resources—social, human, and monetary—and more options to move to greater safety.

The impacts are not limited to Ukraine. Many people around the world have been affected. Refugees from Ukraine have been received by many countries. Many families and communities there opened their homes and offered help. Russia also saw a significant number of people leaving in the wake of the war, particularly young and highly-skilled people trying to escape from the ever-increasing political repression, lack of economic prospects, and, in the case of males, possible army draft. Food supplies from Ukraine's fertile fields have been interrupted, affecting many and contributing to starvation and famine to people in Africa and the Middle East. Russia's weaponization of energy supplies to what it now officially considers "unfriendly countries" of Europe and the West, in general, contributed to rising costs around the world. Upending the post-World War II status quo and causing dramatic shifts in Europe's security landscape, Russia's war brought about a destabilization in several hotspots and heightened political uncertainty and risks on a global scale.

Relational Impact of Sociocultural Trauma

The current experience of the war in Ukraine is interpreted within cultural and historical contexts and, in turn, reinterprets some cultural templates and reshapes identities. Within days after the beginning of the war, the Ukrainian national identity was immensely solidified. Many Ukrainians who previously felt connected to Russia either through family ties or culturally have been distancing themselves from Russianness.

Family connections became a war casualty in both Ukraine and Russia. Since February 24, 2022, many mixed Ukrainian–Russian families have been divided by their stances toward the war. Those under fire in Ukraine tried to share their experience and were disbelieved by their relatives in Russia. As a result, relatives and friends either completely stopped communicating with each other or limited their interactions. This divide happened not only along state lines, but within the Russian society as well. There are multiple accounts of this in the media. (For an example, see independent Russian filmmaker Andrei Loshak's documentary "Broken Ties" on YouTube.)

This represents an immediate and palpable impact of sociocultural trauma on families who live through this experience. But there are also long-term, even transgenerational, consequences of sociocultural traumas, especially when several have been happening over decades. My own acute awareness of living a transgenerational legacy of sociocultural trauma happened many years ago when I (Tatiana) became a mother. I noticed automatic reactions in my parenting, like saying "no" to my then-little daughter when she asked to do something "out of the box." I was very puzzled because I did not have a reason to say "no"—the situation was safe, and rationally I wanted my child to be as free as possible. However, there was something else giving rise to my almost reflexive reactions. That "else" became clearer in my genogram exercise during a counseling program. It stems largely from at least two previous generations of my family living through wars, oppression, and poverty in unstable and dangerous circumstances. Past sociocultural traumas manifested themselves relationally.

The known histories of all nations or communities are marked by social changes and some type of traumatic events. The impacts for the nation and the later assigned meanings of these changes differ. Not all major historical events are traumatic. Some changes and even traumas evoke resilience forces and spark renewal; some lead to serious disturbances of the community and even of the nation. Often both processes take place simultaneously. In this text, we examine what happens to human relationships, including familial ones, during and after the times of big societal changes, and how mental health professionals can respond.

Trauma as a Sociocultural Experience

The term trauma originated from the Greek "injury or wound" and gradually metamorphosed from representing a physical wound first to a psychological one and later to a social phenomenon (see Figley et al., 2017, for a detailed history of the term). Many trauma scholars claim that individual reactions to death and loss that currently would be considered posttraumatic symptoms have been documented since ancient times. However, the phenomenon of psychological trauma became a focus of medical and scholarly attention fairly recently and was itself closely related to societal changes. It has been argued that the Western sociocultural context of the modernity era during the late nineteenth and early twentieth century, with its intense industrial advances, scientific development, and growing interest in an individual, served as a background for attention to psychological consequences of horrific external events on human beings. The further history of describing and formalizing those consequences in diagnostic criteria of posttraumatic disorder is linked to social events of the twentieth century, such as two World Wars and the Vietnam War. While currently the mental health concept of trauma is mostly associated with an individual, attention to societal context is essential in understanding the individual experience of trauma and its relational consequences since its manifestation and interpretation are shaped by culture.

There are various terms used in the literature to describe a life-threatening event in a group's history that impacts not only individual victims but also the entire community—massive trauma, collective trauma, historical trauma, cultural trauma, and social trauma. Studies started with the Holocaust survivors in the mid-1960s (Danieli et al., 2016) but now include many other collective historical traumas such as slavery of and racism towards African-Americans and oppression of Indigenous peoples in North America (Goodman, 2013; Kirmayer et al., 2014). Definitions were introduced in different disciplines and thus have different connotations and associations with particular traumas experienced by a specific group, though they intersect and overlap to some extent. There are multiple debates about conceptualizations of collective trauma (that are not the focus of this book) that reflect the complexity of the phenomenon and a difficulty of finding one inclusive term.

Regardless of a specific term, clinicians have become increasingly aware of the psychological and relational consequences of events at the societal level such as collective violence between groups (genocides, persecutions, war, conflicts, oppression, hate, discrimination) as well as the rapid and radical transformations of the social order that can be considered social traumata. According to Andreas Hamburger (2021), a psychoanalytically oriented clinician and researcher, "the concept of social trauma aims at widening the scope of general clinical theories of posttraumatic disorders by including the specificity of the historical circumstances of their traumatic origin, as well as perpetuating conditions, as seen from history, sociology, and political and cultural science" (p. 6).

Sociologists consider the impact of such events on a particular society as possible cultural trauma that can be broadly defined as "an invasive and overwhelming event that is believed to undermine or overwhelm one or several essential ingredients of a culture or the culture as a whole" (Smelser, 2004, p. 38). One of the principal aspects of cultural trauma conceptualization is a process of social construction. Not all big, or even traumatic in the sense of negative impact, events become collective traumas. Trauma is interpreted within the societal and cultural contexts and, consequently, may be different for different cultural groups in a given society.

In this book, we use the term "sociocultural trauma" to highlight the following aspects: (1) the cause of trauma is from and within the social context; (2) the impact depends on the social location of groups, families, and individuals; (3) trauma is interpreted within societal and cultural contexts, and in this regard is socially constructed; and (4) in its turn, social traumatic experience impacts culture. This trauma refers to historical events and ongoing injustice, either large- or small scale, that had a destructive impact on people's lives and well-being or societal structures and organization. It includes not only wars or genocides but also traumatic societal changes, such as the radical transformation of the social system, including the fall of the communist system – the historical event particularly relevant to the countries of Eastern Europe. The impact of such trauma on culture is important. While culture, as a foundational fabric of our social existence, is sometimes clearly visible, for example, in ways of communicating or in attire signaling one's cultural identity, it is often not immediately visible. Sociocultural trauma may be reflected in deeply held values and beliefs that serve as scripts for everyday behaviors and practices and are passed on from generation to generation. The effect of sociocultural trauma on individual and relational well-being involves these ongoing reciprocal influences.

Model of Sociocultural Trauma

Conceptualization of a complex phenomenon, such as sociocultural trauma, requires an integrative and multisystemic approach to avoid simplistic and reductionistic understanding. Our model (Fig. 1.1), "The impact of sociocultural trauma on relational well-being," is modified from Sztompka's (2004) representation of the sequence of trauma at the societal level to include relational aspects of sociocultural trauma. While not intended to be a fully comprehensive theory of sociocultural trauma or its impact on human relations, this conceptualization serves as a possible foundation for addressing the complex nature of ongoing nonlinear processes that may, and most likely do, include the simultaneous presence and interactions of opposite processes, such as traumatization and growth, identity loss, and identity formation at both societal (the top level in Fig. 1.1) and personal levels (the lower level in Fig. 1.1). The word "trauma" has been used (and defined in Webster) to convey several meanings—a traumatic event, experience of that event, injury or impact of that event, and sequelae or consequences of that impact. To differentiate between those meanings, we use the terms "traumatogenic event", "traumatic event", or "traumata" to represent sociohistorical events and "trauma" to represent the ongoing effects on people, their relationships, communities, and societies.

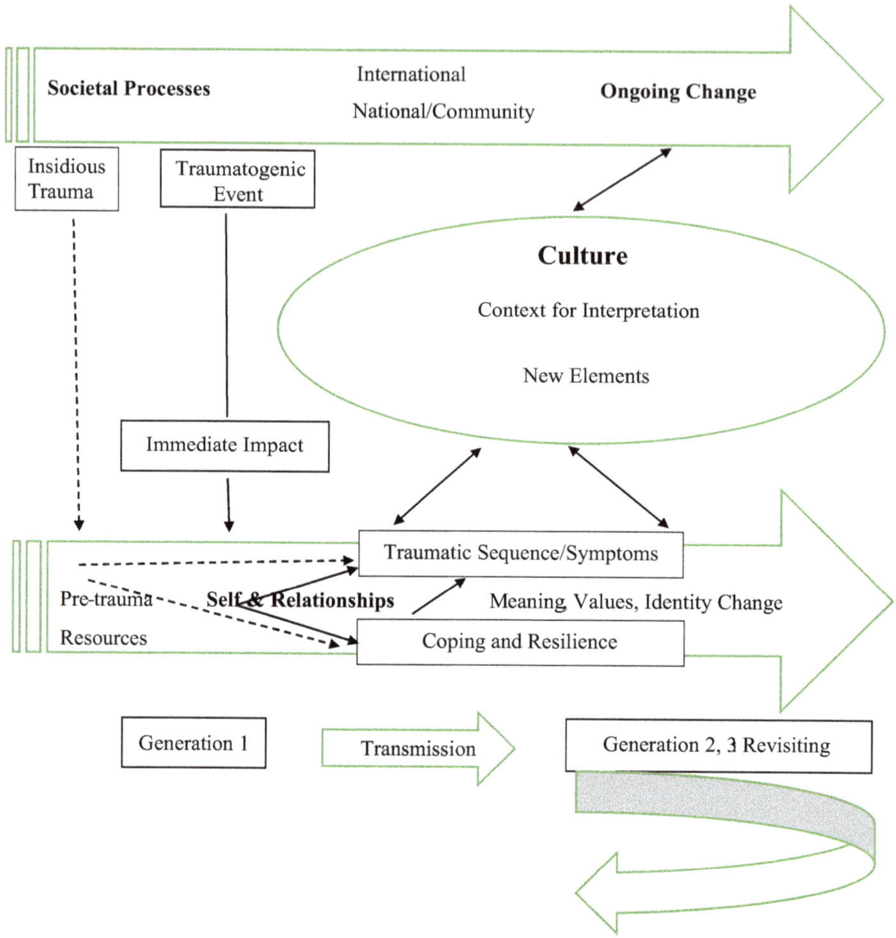

Fig. 1.1 The impact of sociocultural trauma on relational well-being

Time is an essential dimension for understanding traumas at individual, relational, and societal levels. As Killian (2016) stressed, trauma disrupts "the unifying thread of temporality". In the mental health field, there has been a distinction between acute trauma, associated with an isolated event, such as rape, and chronic trauma associated with prolonged, continuing events, such as domestic abuse. Most definitions of trauma, both individual and social, imply clearly identifiable and finite events, even though they last for several years or decades. However, some societal processes, such as social oppression and discrimination are ongoing. Hardy (2019) conceptualized poverty as sociocultural trauma and asserted that "… all manifestations of oppression, whether racial, gender, or class, represent forms of trauma" (p. 58). Brown (2017) provided examples of "insidious traumatization," the term introduced by Root (1992), experienced by members of socially marginalized groups whose everyday life is full of reminders of the potential for trauma exposure or the absence of safety and protection. The impact and long-term effects of insidious traumatization were illustrated by Brown (2017) with the metaphor of small drops of acid falling on a stone:

> Each drop by itself does little damage and in fact may etch the stone in such [a]way as to make it more beautiful. Thus, in some ways, the experience of daily microaggressions may evoke resilient coping responses; humor and ritual in many target groups can be conceived of as protective strategies for dealing with both actual and insidious threat. Despite all efforts at coping, each drop of emotional acid creates just enough damage to render the next drop more damaging. Over time, a fissure develops in the form of an emotional vulnerability that is invisible as long as a certain degree of environmental homeostasis is maintained. (p. 509)

In our model of the impact of sociocultural trauma on well-being, we included an acute, one-time traumatogenic event (the solid vertical line) as well as chronic processes of insidious traumatization (the dotted vertical line). If we follow the historical process of extrapolating existing individual diagnoses or phenomena of trauma to the social level, then we can say that some groups or nations experienced complex trauma, which refers to the experience of repeated, simultaneous, or consecutive traumatogenic events of various nature during a relatively long period of time. When waves from different sources of social shocks or traumata interface, then very complex aftereffects can be produced. This is especially relevant to situations in Eastern Europe with its history of multiple life-changing social events.

In determining the effects of sociocultural trauma on psychological and relational well-being, individual and interpersonal realities are hardly separable. "Self" exists and develops within relationships. Self-identities are formed through social interactions. Traumatic experience impacts both individuals and their relational "net", such as families, friends, peers, and, more broadly, other humans. Its effects are determined by complex and cumulative effects of risk and protective factors in all systems – individual, biological and psychological, familial, cultural, communal, national, and international. The same historical event, even within the same larger culture, may have different consequences for people from different backgrounds and of different social locations. The actual immediate impact and consequences will depend on the pre-trauma situation in terms of resources or disadvantages as well as the person or group's social location within the larger social system.

Trauma experts in different fields underline that severe traumatic experience shakes the fundamental conception of the world and human relations. Summarizing the existential psychology perspective on trauma Reuther (2017) stated, "The aftermath of trauma may result in myriad debilitating cognitive, behavioral, emotional, and physiological symptoms, but it is critically important to consider the profound impact trauma has on the lived experience of the whole person as a being in the world" (p. 535). Different cultures and societies historically hold different worldviews about the importance of happiness or suffering in human life, whether the environment—"the world"—is safe or just, and whether other humans are trustworthy. Man-made disasters and interpersonal violence either confirm or decrease beliefs that the world is safe and people, or some groups of people, can be trusted. One of the consequences of sociocultural trauma is the demolition of "basic trust," which is an essential component of all enduring social relationships and human agency (Sztompka, 2000).

Response to historical trauma or other severe adversities may produce not only destructive or negative effects but also evoke new ways of adaptation, stimulate growth, and create new meanings. Walsh (2016) emphasized, "Resilience entails more than managing stressful conditions, shouldering a burden, or surviving an ordeal. It involves the potential for personal and relational transformation and positive growth that can be forged out of adversity" (p. 315). Resilience can be manifested at any systemic level—individual, familial, communal, and national, as well as at their intersections. Resilience forces in one system may enhance and stimulate or counteract another. The factors affecting family resilience in the face of sociocultural trauma are contextual and depend on each family's values and beliefs, communication styles, structural and relational resources, and particular life challenges (Walsh, 2016). These processes are not static; they change over time, and families evolve.

Time is needed to process trauma, heal, and evolve. For families, time includes generational processes. The concept of transgenerational/intergenerational transmission of trauma has been applied to and studied for various types of trauma, including collective and historical ones (Kirmayer et al., 2014). This process is not always (or probably never) a linear one, such as a direct transmission of posttraumatic symptoms from parents to children, but rather a complex one, with each generation dealing with trauma and its effects in its own way. In the qualitative study of three generations of Holocaust survivors in Israel, Chaitin (2002) concluded that dealing with the Holocaust was important for all of three generations but posed different challenges for each. Porobić (2021) described generational differences in dealing with the past in Germany where "… only the third generation that was able to vocalise the guilt of Nazi crimes committed during World War II" (p. 256).

Generational differences in processing traumatic experience can partly be explained by changing societal contexts and an evolving cultural milieu. New generations, raised under different conditions in a reformed society, often clash with cultural legacies and traditions that reflect traumatogenic experience of prior generations (Sztompka, 2004). On the other hand, sometimes the effect of the trauma on collective meaning may increase over time, as focus shifts from the immediacy of personal loss to long-term "lessons" groups construct regarding the traumatic event (Hirschberger, 2018). These collective representations of the traumatic event(s) become embedded as a pivotal element of social identity (Porobić, 2021) and may lead to social cohesion or division. Volkan's (2021) concept of the "chosen trauma" and "chosen glory" describes possible long-lasting effects of ancestral traumas due to ethnic, national, religious, racial, or political ideological conflicts for large-group identities, which can be reactivated during current conflicts. Generational differences in processing traumatic experience partly can be explained by changing societal context, including at national and international levels, and cultural norms.

The framework for understanding the effects of sociocultural trauma presented in this chapter shows that the cause of trauma originated in the larger social system, and the experience is embedded in complex historical, social, and cultural contexts that change over time. Understanding the complex and cumulative effects of risk and protective factors in any particular situation involves examining and addressing systemic intersections—individual, biological and psychological, familial, cultural, communal, national, and international. While this framework can be applied in any setting, in this book we focus on the Eastern European context.

Eastern European Historical Context of Trauma

The Eastern European countries share massive historical traumatic events that shook Europe in the twentieth century, in particular, the tragedies of the two World Wars and the Holocaust. However, the Eastern European region also has its unique history related to the establishment of communist regimes and their subsequent falls, with transitions to state independence for some countries, and radical transformations in political and economic structures. Even the term "Eastern European" is not purely geographical but has geopolitical, cultural, and socioeconomic allusions and is defined differently by various experts. One of the definitions, often questioned and disputed, is based on the East–West divide in Europe during the Cold War and refers to the former communist European states. By this definition, Hungary, Romania, Moldova, and Serbia, located geographically in central and southeastern parts of Europe, can be considered "Eastern European." In this section we present a very brief overview of the twentieth-century historical events in the region. However, within the region each society has unique ways of dealing with the consequences of those pivotal historical events and their experience of sociocultural trauma.

As already noted above, the term Eastern Europe is imprecise and politically contested. However, for the purposes of this book it seems a reasonable term of convenience since the countries in focus, while maintaining their distinct sociocultural identities, shared the twentieth-century tectonic historical shifts that affected their societies and historical trajectories in a fundamental way and certainly inflicted several major traumatic events. These events were arguably unrivaled in their magnitude and impact for the world in general, but Europe and especially Eastern Europe in particular.

Some of the initial tremors could be felt in the Russo-Japanese war of 1905, which ended in Russia's defeat, and the subsequent first Russian revolution, which, while unsuccessful, shook the foundations of the Russian Empire. World War I of 1914–1918 was the first dramatic shock that forever changed the face of Europe. Two of the empires and their centuries-old monarchies, Russian and Austro-Hungarian, that most of our selected countries, with the exception of Serbia, were a part of, collapsed (see Maps A.1 and A.2, Appendix, this volume). Human losses were immense (one should bear in mind that numbers of war casualties, as well as victims of Russia's internal repressions vary widely, and given the range, conservative estimates were mostly used for this book): at least 3.3 million military and civilian deaths combined for Russia, 1.4 million for Austria-Hungary, 550 thousand for Serbia, and 525 thousand for Romania, with millions more wounded and captured or missing (Prost, 2014). Russia and particularly Hungary suffered huge territorial losses—Poland and Finland broke away from Russia, while the Trianon treaty of 1920 deprived Hungary of roughly two-thirds of its territories (compare Maps A.1 and A.2, Appendix, this volume) and population, with about three million ethnic Hungarians ending up outside its borders (Zeidler, 2014). The war brought destruction and economic ruin to most of Europe. Russia's October revolution of 1917 resulted in the world's first communist regime. In its wake, foreign intervention and Civil War followed. They lasted until 1922 and led to hunger, mass poverty, and more horrible loss of human life, which actually exceeded Russia's World War I toll, with the total number so outrageous that Guinness World Records (n.d.) lists it as the world's highest death toll from a civil war at 1.5 million combatants and eight million civilian population dead. Other countries also experienced significant postwar social upheaval.

Russia then continued with the radical communist socioeconomic experiment, which, while lifting the country out of economic backwardness and destruction, proved to be extremely traumatic in terms of human price. In less than two decades between the world wars, the Soviet Union, which replaced the old Russia (see Maps A.2, Appendix, this volume), experienced Stalin's brutal internal policies, such as, among others, the forced collectivization of agriculture, the establishment of a notorious system of forced labor camps (GULAG), the Holodomor (mass famine engineered through the confiscation of grains) in Ukraine, and the extensive political repressions culminating in the Great Purge of 1937–1938. While the exact total number of victims has been hard, and may be impossible, to establish, there is no doubt that it runs in millions of lives.

World War II of 1939–1945 put Eastern Europe right in the epicenter of another massive wave of destruction and suffering again. The losses remain unparalleled in human history—the Soviet Union lost approximately 26.6 million people (Interfax, 2015), Yugoslavia, of which Serbia was the biggest and most populous part—1.0 million, Romania—833 thousand, and Hungary—580 thousand (The National WWII Museum, n.d.). Millions more were wounded, and millions were homeless. Economy lay in ruins.

While the remainder of the century was never this horrifically brutal again, there was no lack of further turbulence and traumatic events. Mired in the grip of the Cold War, most of the countries of Eastern Europe ended up in the totalitarian communist camp dominated by the USSR (Map A.3, Appendix, this volume). Any attempt to shake off Soviet control or adopt a measure of democracy was put down by force, as in 1956 in Hungary and 1968 in Czechoslovakia. Internal dissent was repressed. Eastern European countries went through the nationalization of economy, and private entrepreneurship was for the most part outlawed. The peoples of Eastern Europe had to adjust to the new economic system. That state-dominated system, while guaranteeing basic social services, proved to be economically inefficient and eventually led to the gradual stagnation and deterioration of living standards, especially when compared to the dynamically developing post-War Western Europe. The Soviet Union was particularly affected as it was increasingly unable to ensure economic growth and prosperity under the crushing burden of military expenses. This situation was further exacerbated by its military involvement in Afghanistan in 1979, which led to a decade of an unsuccessful war with a high human toll. Ultimately the whole system became untenable, and with the arrival of perestroika in the Soviet Union in the late 1980s and the weakening of Soviet political, economic, and military control over Eastern Europe, the formerly socialist Eastern Europe countries were able to set themselves free from repressive communist rule.

The USSR itself was dissolved in late 1991, and the Cold War finally ended (see Map A.4, Appendix, this volume, for eventual national borders changes and their current state). However, the transition to democracy and free-market economy proved to be a significant stress, and the collapse of the USSR and Yugoslavia brought about military conflicts resulting in hundreds of thousands of dead—Transnistria in Moldova, Chechnya in Russia, and an extremely violent and bloody break-up of Yugoslavia with Serbia involved in hostilities with its neighbors and its eventual bombing by NATO in 1999. Economically and socially, there was a lot of suffering for most people, especially at the initial stage, as economies were privatized, inefficient companies closed or sold and restructured, jobs eliminated, and social expenses curtailed. Even after all these years, the consequences of these continuous dramatic societal transformations are still felt deeply by many countries and their people. Russia's resurgent imperialism and unwarranted aggression against Ukraine in 2022 led to heavy loss of life, a severe economic blow to Ukraine (but also, due to Western sanctions, to Russia's economy), and put a lot of pressure on the whole region, which is helping Ukraine in military, economic, and humanitarian terms. As of the time of writing, the fighting continues to rage without any immediate prospect of peace in sight. However, one thing looks certain—the already huge number of families and people directly affected and heavily traumatized by this war, particularly among Ukrainians, will likely grow much higher.

Clinical Implications

The personal and relational well-being of Eastern Europeans and those with family roots or other connections from this region is inevitably related to the historical contexts described above, as these legacies interact with current lived experience, developmental processes, family and community interactions, and evolving sociocultural norms and expectations. Naming these contexts and the likelihood of sociocultural trauma is important not just for the sake of creating another word or concept but for the sake of action. Acknowledgment of this phenomenon is needed for a healing process, both at a societal level as a justice reparation and in clinical practice as a legitimate and important focus of treatment. While the impact on individuals and even on communities has been well documented, the complex consequences of sociocultural traumas on relationships have been less explored, especially in the Eastern European context. This is an important topic for systemic family therapists and other clinicians.

Our Collective Work

We invited systemic therapists and researchers from five Eastern European countries—Hungary, Russia, Romania, Moldova, and Serbia—to contribute to this volume. Each author presents background about their country, their national experience of sociocultural trauma, and its impact on interpersonal relationships across various social locations and national or ethnic identities within the current social–cultural–economic–political contexts. Their perspectives and interpretations are influenced and informed by their professional and personal backgrounds, experiences, and positions. Though no one view can be fully comprehensive or "objective," this collective work provides some understanding of relational dynamics and examples of the lived experience of individuals and families in these Eastern European countries, as well as recommendations for clinical practice.

The final two chapters help readers expand beyond these five countries. Chapter 7 uses Boszormenyi-Nagy's contextual therapy to address the legacies of sociocultural trauma when working with issues such as immigration, couple dynamics, parenting, and communication. Chapter 8 draws on conclusions from Eastern European experience in previous chapters to offer an overall framework for clinical practice that assesses the effects of sociocultural trauma and attends to the nuances and complexities of how these may differentially impact people across diverse contexts and situations.

We invite readers to engage from their own sociocultural position. Like Tatiana and the other chapter authors, many of you have personal familiarity with life in Eastern Europe. The information on sociocultural trauma presented here captures and names some of your experiences. Others, like me (Carmen), may never have been to countries featured in this book. I joined Tatiana in writing this chapter and editing this book out of my interest in family therapy and the day-to-day impact of larger societal contexts on people's lives. There are many Eastern European immigrants in my city and nearby communities. Some have been my clients; some have been my students. I learned from them, but I am chagrined regarding how superficial my knowledge of Eastern European life has been. And, I have never directly suffered the consequences of war or political oppression. Working with Tatiana on this project, which unexpectedly is happening during the invasion of Ukraine, has been eye-opening. I am grateful to glimpse into her family's life and into the lives of those shared by the authors of this book. I hope all of you will leave your journey through these varied chapters personally and professionally richer and inspired.

References

Brown, L. (2017). Contributions of feminist and critical psychologies to trauma psychology. In S. N. Gold (Editor-in-Chief), *APA handbook of trauma psychology: Vol. 1. Foundations in knowledge* (pp. 501–526). American Psychological Association. https://doi.org/10.1037/0000019-025.

Chaitin, J. (2002). Issues and interpersonal values among three generations in families of Holocaust survivors. *Journal of Social and Personal Relationships, 19*(3), 379–402. https://doi.org/10.1177/0265407502193005
Danieli, Y., Norris, F. H., & Engdahl, B. (2016). Multigenerational legacies of trauma: Modeling the what and how of transmission. *American Journal of Orthopsychiatry, 86*(6), 639–651. https://doi.org/10.1037/ort0000145
Figley, C. R., Amy E. Ellis, Reuther, B. T., & Gold, S. N. (2017). The study of trauma: A historical overview. In S. N. Gold (Editor-in-Chief), *APA handbook of trauma psychology: Vol. 1. Foundations in knowledge* (pp. 1–11). American Psychological Association. https://doi.org/10.1037/0000019-001.
Goodman, R. D. (2013). The transgenerational trauma and resilience genogram. *Counselling Psychology Quarterly, 26*(3–4), 386–405. https://doi.org/10.1080/09515070.2013.820172
Guinness World Records. (n.d.). *Highest death toll from a civil war.* https://www.guinnessworldrecords.com/world-records/highest-death-toll-from-a-civil-war
Hamburger, A. (2021). Social trauma: A bridging concept. In A. Hamburger, C. Hancheva, & V. D. Volkan (Eds.), *Social trauma—An interdisciplinary textbook* (pp. 3–16). Springer. https://doi.org/10.1007/978-3-030-47817-9
Hardy, K. V. (2019). The sociocultural trauma of poverty: Theoretical and clinical considerations for working with poor families. In M. McGoldrick & K. V. Hardy (Eds.), *Re-visioning family therapy: Addressing diversity in clinical practice* (3rd ed., pp. 57–72). The Guilford Press.
Hirschberger, G. (2018). Collective trauma and the social construction of meaning. *Frontiers in Psychology, 9*, 1441. https://doi.org/10.3389/fpsyg.2018.01441
Interfax (2015, November 13). *The Ministry of Defense clarified the losses of the USSR in the Great Patriotic War.* Interfax.ru. https://www.interfax.ru/russia/479070
Killian, K. D. (2016). Time, trauma, and ambiguous loss: Working with families with missing members in postconflict Cyprus. In L. L. Charlés & G. Samarasinghe (Eds.), *Family therapy in global humanitarian contexts: Voices and issues from the field* (pp. 77–89). Springer Science + Business Media.
Kirmayer, L. J., Gone, J. P., & Moses, J. (2014). Rethinking historical trauma. *Transcultural Psychiatry, 51*(3), 299–319. https://doi.org/10.1177/1363461514536358
McGoldrick, M. (2019). Homelessness and the spiritual meaning of home. In M. McGoldrick & K. V. Hardy (Eds.), *Re-visioning family therapy: Addressing diversity in clinical practice* (3rd ed., pp. 93–107). The Guilford Press.
Porobić, S. (2021). Social identity transformations and social trauma nexus. In A. Hamburger, C. Hancheva, & V. D. Volkan (Eds.), *Social trauma – An interdisciplinary textbook* (pp. 253–260). Springer. https://doi.org/10.1007/978-3-030-47817-9_26
Prost, A. (2014, October 8). War losses. In U. Daniel, P. Gatrell, O. Janz, H. Jones, J. Keene, A. Kramer, & B. Nasson (Eds.), *1914–1918-online. International encyclopedia of the first world war.* Freie Universität Berlin. https://doi.org/10.15463/ie1418.10271
Reuther, B. T. (2017). Philosophical and existential perspectives on trauma. In S. N. Gold (Editor-in-Chief), *APA handbook of trauma psychology: Vol. 1. Foundations in knowledge* (pp. 527–545). American Psychological Association. https://doi.org/10.1037/0000019-026.
Root, M. P. P. (1992). Reconstructing the impact of trauma on personality. In L. S. Brown & M. Ballou (Eds.), *Personality and psychopathology: Feminist reappraisals* (pp. 229–265). The Guilford Press.
Smelser, N. J. (2004). Psychological trauma and cultural trauma. In J. C. Alexander, R. Eyerman, B. Giesen, N. J. Smelser, & P. Sztompka (Eds.), *Cultural trauma and collective identity* (pp. 31–59). University of California Press.
Sztompka, P. (2000). *Trust: A sociological theory.* Cambridge University Press.
Sztompka, P. (2004). The trauma of social change: A case of postcommunist societies. In J. C. Alexander, R. Eyerman, B. Giesen, N. J. Smelser, & P. Sztompka (Eds.), *Cultural trauma and collective identity* (pp. 155–195). University of California Press.

The National WWII Museum. (n.d.). *Worldwide deaths in World War II*.https://www.nationalww2museum.org/students-teachers/student-resources/research-starters/research-starters-worldwide-deaths-world-war

Volkan, V. D. (2021). Chosen traumas and their impact on current political/societal conflicts. In A. Hamburger, C. Hancheva, & V. D. Volkan (Eds.), *Social trauma – An interdisciplinary textbook* (pp. 17–24). Springer. https://doi.org/10.1007/978-3-030-47817-9_2

Walsh, F. (2016). Family resilience: A developmental systems framework. *European Journal of Developmental Psychology, 13*(3), 313–324. https://doi.org/10.1080/17405629.2016.1154035

Zeidler, M. (2014, October 8). Trianon, treaty of. In U. Daniel, P. Gatrell, O. Janz, H. Jones, J. Keene, A. Kramer, & B. Nasson (Eds.), *1914–1918-online. International encyclopedia of the first world war*. Freie Universität Berlin. https://doi.org/10.15463/ie1418.10033

Chapter 2
When History Hits Home: Historical Intergenerational Trauma and Hope in Hungary

Emőke Tarján, Patrik Pál Wächter, and Tamás Wittmann

> *A person's life is never the life of one person only, it is always the life of a country, a world, an era.*
>
> *—Magda Szabó (1983, p. 13)*

We begin by sharing our personal contexts and how they connect to the contextual approach to sociocultural trauma we describe in this chapter.

Emőke Tarján

I am a doctor, psychiatrist, psychotherapist, and family therapist. I work with individuals, couples, and families in private practice. As the head of a family-systems therapy training program, I train future family therapists. I have experienced the destructive effects of historical and political traumas at both personal and professional levels. Born in 1960 and growing up in a family of doctors and teachers, my family tried to protect me from the humiliation and isolation that characterized the Kádár-era and the discrimination that threatened the children of the "class-alien" intellectual families. Yet, I can still recall how petrified I felt on Mondays as a 6-year-old whom the teacher could ask whether I had been to church the day before.

Translated by Orsolya Wächter-Szili

E. Tarján (✉) · T. Wittmann
Family Systems Therapy Institute, Budapest, Hungary

P. P. Wächter
The National Archives of Hungary, Szombathely, Hungary

T. Glebova, C. Knudson-Martin (eds.), *Sociocultural Trauma and Well-Being in Eastern European Family Therapy*, AFTA SpringerBriefs in Family Therapy,
https://doi.org/10.1007/978-3-031-29995-7_2

My parents had prepared me: when asked this question, I had to lie, the answer was "no." Had I told the truth, I would have been made to stand in front of my class and called a stupid, ignorant child—mislead by her stupid, ignorant parents who taught her to believe in God instead of communist ideas and values. Thanks to my parents' "preparation for survival," I managed to avoid this humiliation. However, I developed a gut-level feeling of fear and shame (and so did a great part of my generation) when I have to show my true self and talk about deep and personal feelings, emotions, and values.

These experiences explain why it is such a challenge, at the same time a wonderful opportunity, for me to be a co-author of this chapter, and—together with my colleagues—write about the past, present, and future of the Hungarian people. Doing so brings me back to my most motivating goals: to improve the quality of life for my family, my loved ones, and my patients, and thus for the coming generations.

After completing my studies at the medical university, I worked in a psychiatry ward with people with psychotic and other psychological disorders, and later, as a psychotherapist, with individuals, couples, and families in outpatient care. I can hardly recall a case where the past did not come up. I always started the process with the patient's own past. The longer I had been in my profession, the further back in time we delved, looking at the life of the parents, then the grandparents, their circumstances, and the historical and political contexts among which the ancestors had to live—at times only surviving. Often they could not be good enough parents because all they could do was stay alive. I came to understand that present symptoms often originate in old unprocessed events. The contextual approach of Iván Böszörményi-Nagy (1984/2013) was of great help and became a guideline for me both in my profession and my personal life.

Most of my patients are Hungarians aged 35–55. Their parents and grandparents, who grew up during the communist dictatorship, learned how to keep secrets, hide and protect their values, and obscure communication for the sake of survival—open communication would have been fatal for them—to be suspicious at all times, and even to deny family values. Yet, these survival mechanisms had not always been sufficient to protect them and their children. In the meantime, the political system changed, the dictatorship ended, and democracy was introduced in 1990. The old means of defense, which were life-saving during the times of dictatorship, became outdated, harmful ways of conduct in the democracy. Thus, we were left with dysfunctional behavior. The symptoms which come to surface in my office today most often hide the unprocessed suffering of previous generations—unfair deaths, tortures, the ungrieved dead, dread of political retaliation, and countless means of self-defense which may have ensured survival for a while, but later gave grounds to dysfunctional behavior, sickness, and unhappiness. Our task is to place their symptoms in a contextual framework and take it into consideration when making clinical assessment and conceptualization. We must be familiar with the cruel circumstances that affected the families of the twentieth century.

Patrik Pál Wächter

I was born in 1981 toward the end of the communist regime. I completed an MA in History and worked as a history teacher for 7 years. I currently work at the National Archives of Hungary where I research crimes committed by occupying Soviet troops in 1945. Besides history, I have always been interested in psychology and have participated in family-systems therapy training programs. During one of the training sessions, I realized how these two disciplines (history and family-systems therapy) are connected in the effect of historical traumas on families. I have memories from my childhood during the time of state socialism. Even as a child I knew that I should not speak about certain things outside of our home because if I did, my parents could have gotten into trouble. My parents, as well as my grandparents, were all persecuted to some extent by the communists. The result was fear and forced silence, which harmed our family life in many ways. According to contextual theory, I belong to the third generation, which has the opportunity to complete the repayment, as described by Böszörményi-Nagy (1984). This is one of the reasons I feel so motivated to be a part of this project.

Tamás Wittmann

I was born in 1992, after the political change that ended communist government in Hungary. My generation has no direct experience about the most horrible times of twentieth-century Hungarian history; our knowledge comes from historical resources and stories. Since we were born into a free, democratic world, I believe it is both our right and obligation to talk openly about the burdens of our past and face the unprocessed trauma of our families and our country. Not only is it an opportunity, but also our responsibility to help our society by talking about the past, bringing up the pain our society has gone through, and taking an active part in healing the wounds. This is the reason I studied psychology, specialized in social psychology, then started to deal with family systems therapy. Currently, I am a PhD student in geopolitics. My field of research is the identity and political environment of Hungarian national minorities living in those areas that were detached from Hungary during the course of the twentieth century.

Brief Overview of Hungary

Hungary is a country with a history of more than 1000 years, located in Eastern-Central Europe. The population in 2020 was approximately 9,770,000; the area is 35,920 square miles (about the size of Indiana). Based on data from the 2011 census, the main ethnicities are 85.6% Hungarian, 3.2% Roma, and 1.9% German; Hungarian is the mother tongue for 98.9% of the population. Concerning religious affiliation, 54.3% of the population are Christians, 0.1% Jewish, 0.1% Muslims, and the rest have no religious affiliations or did not answer (KSH, 2013).

The GDP per capita was $32,600 in 2019 and $31,000 in 2020, which ranks 63rd in the world. Hungary is a member of the UNO, NATO, the European Union, the OECD, the World Bank, the Schengen area, and along with Poland, Czechia (formerly the Czech Republic), and Slovakia, a founding member of the Visegrád Group, a cultural, economic, political, and diplomatic alliance of Central-European countries (CIA, 2022). On the Human Development Index (HDI), which measures life expectancy, literacy, education, and standard of living, Hungary ranked 46th in 2021, with a "very high" score of 0.846 (Human Development Reports, 2022). In 2020, according to the Global Gender Gap Index, out of 158 countries Hungary came 100th with a score of 0.688 concerning equal rights for women—mostly pulled down by the low participation rate of women in politics (World Economic Forum, 2021). A year later, Hungary moved ahead six places on this list, and the first female president of the country took her office this year, which may help further improve this process.

According to WHO data, Hungary's suicide rate in 2019 was 11.8 in 100,000, which brings Hungary to the 54th place worldwide (World Health Organization, 2021). This number was considerably higher in 2016 (22.2), and for a long time the country was among the top 20 worldwide. Even though the figures show significant improvement, this ratio is still very high, leaving Hungary in the top third on the list of countries, and giving a reflection of the mental health of Hungarians. In 2019, 41.5% of the population aged 15 or over were moderate drinkers and 10.8% were excessive drinkers; thus, alcohol abuse is characteristic of Hungarians (KSH, 2020). The leading causes of death are malignant tumors, responsible for 22.4% of all deaths in 2020 (KSH, 2022a).

The population growth rate was −0.29% in 2021, and the total fertility rate is 1.48 child/woman. As of this writing, life expectancy is 73.27 years for men and 80.83 years for women (CIA, 2022). The number of marriages almost doubled between 2014 and 2021, while the number of divorces has continuously been declining for the last 15 years (KSH, 2022b). After Hungary joined the European Union in 2004, a strong wave of emigration to Western Europe started. Along with the natural decline of the population, this poses considerable economic threat to our society. The tendency changed in 2018, when the number of people returning to Hungary became higher than the number of emigrants. In 2020, the ratio was 23,104 returning citizens for 19,322 emigrants (KSH, 2022c).

Historical Background

The origin of the Hungarian people is obscure. Scientific proofs of the various hypotheses change frequently (Molnár, 2001). The Hungarian tribes moved to the Carpathian basin at the end of the ninth century. Around 1000 AD, the first king, St. Stephen, integrated the country into medieval Christian Europe by adapting its administrative, religious, and cultural patterns. The Hungarian Kingdom in this integral form came to an end after a fatal defeat by the Ottomans in 1526, followed by the occupation of its territories, and has never been fully restored to its previous independent and integrated status. During the wars of the following centuries, significant areas were destroyed and depopulated. After the country was taken back from the Ottomans, the area was repopulated with other ethnic groups. The main focus of the Hungarian political elite was on the attempt to restore the "former glory" of the Hungarian Kingdom through wars of independence or via compromises with the Habsburg royal dynasty in power. However, the other ethnic groups living in the territory of Hungary saw these attempts as suppressive, imperialistic, and limiting conduct. This process continued until the end of World War I.

The loss of World War I was followed by troubled years of red-and-white terror that meant a huge trauma for the society. The Peace Treaty of Trianon of 1920 shocked our nation: 2/3 of the former territory of Hungary was lost (compare Maps A.1 and A.2, Appendix, this volume), and 1/3 of Hungarians—about three million people—became citizens of other countries against their own will, causing frustration for the Hungarians, creating an unstable region, and providing a basis for further ethnic conflicts. We could hardly find a family in Hungary that was not affected by the Trianon Peace Treaty in some way. They were forced to leave their homes and escape or became victims in other ways. The demand for revision of the territorial losses drove the country into World War II, which—besides the general losses and traumas of war—resulted in Nazi occupation and the Holocaust, followed by Soviet occupation and the deportation of hundreds of thousands of people. (See Boxes 1 and 2 on the timeline, Fig. 2.1.)

After World War II, the borders of the Trianon Peace Treaty were reestablished. In accordance with the Yalta Agreement, Hungary became part of the sphere of influence of the Soviet Union. The Hungarians were hoping for the creation of a democratic state, but due to Moscow's orders, the building of a Stalinist dictatorship was started in 1948 with Mátyás Rákosi as a leader.

On October 23, 1956, a revolution broke out to oppose the almost one decade of communist dictatorship and 12 years of Soviet occupation. The main demands included withdrawal of the Soviet military troops, penalizing the dictators, and ensuring liberties. For a few days, it seemed like the impossible had been achieved, but it soon turned out that Hungary did not stand a chance. The prime minister declared Hungary neutral, but none of the great powers ensured this. The revolution was crushed and the Soviet army stayed in Hungary for 35 more years.

Between the 1960s and 1990s keeping silent was crucial, and in return the Hungarians were granted an acceptable standard of living among the Eastern

Bloc—all we had to do was deny the faith and deeds of our ancestors. Generations were raised in a way that things could not be called what they actually were but had to be lied about. The Peace Treaty of Trianon, the revolution of 1956, and even the Holocaust were not to be talked about. Many Nazi victimizers became victimizers in the communist regime, and people could easily fall victim to political systems of two extremes. Religious people were class-aliens, subject to ridicule, discrimination, and persecution. The system under János Kádár aimed at forming a Marxist-socialist society; however, all they managed to achieve was creating new inequalities in the place of the old ones: "political position replacing possessions, labor organization membership instead of personal property" (Valuch, 2002). The state controlled and regulated the private lives of its citizens via enforcement, secret police, and an extensive network of spies. As a result, personal and family histories were re-evaluated, mistrust developed between people, even between the closest friends, that ultimately led to the total vulnerability of the individuals. This time period is referred to as the Kádár-era after the political leader János Kádár. For further traumatizing events, see Box 3 in the timeline (Fig. 2.1).

The political change in 1990 brought about unemployment and the tribulations of transition because of the privatization and the introduction of a free market economy. The state of ownership was not restored to what it had been prior to the collectivization of 1948, and only partial compensation took place. There was no impeachment of the politicians who took part in the crimes of the communist system. The dream of generations about freedom turned into bitter disappointment.

Between 1918–1990 the practice of power—constitutional, or unconstitutional, even violent form of state—changed nine times. This in itself inevitably brought about an immense amount of trauma, family tragedies, and oppositions and resulted in people taking a passive attitude as a form of self-defense and abstinence from politics (as one could easily be executed for taking an active role in the previous political system). The communist system in rule until 1990 was patronizing, yet intolerant toward anything individual, which extinguished responsibility and initiative in most people. Instead, we were left with silence, secrets, and collaboration in return for advantages, or a martyr's role, passivity, scapegoating, and lack of responsibility or solution-seeking attitude, the effects of which can still be felt both at the individual and the societal level.

Healing Political–Historical Transgenerational Trauma

According to the relational ethics of the contextual approach, human relationships are generally characterized by a balance of give and take, entitlement, and commitment that connect generations. When out of balance, this heritage may be a destructive one, "entitling" the descendants to destructive behavior toward others or themselves. They pass on what they received. If the parents are subject to unfair suffering by destructive external political–historical forces, the descendants will be bound by a stronger loyalty to previous generations—a process of which they are

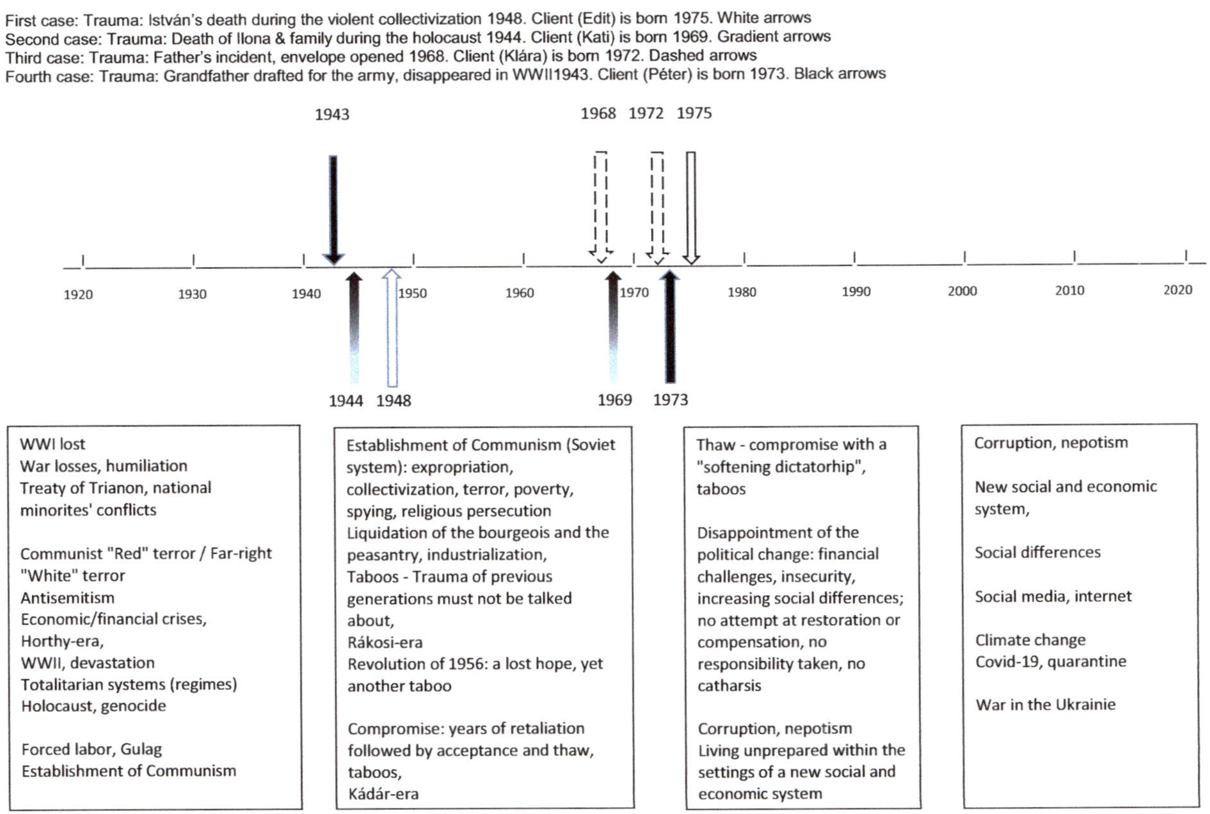

Above: social traumas in Hungary in the course of the past 100 years. The events follow a chronological order and are marked parallel to the timeline of the cases described.

Fig. 2.1 Social traumas in Hungary in the course of the past 100 years

often unaware. This hinders the process of individuation from the parents, and destructive entitlement may strengthen. This phenomenon is called destructive loyalty (Böszörményi-Nagy, 1984/2013). The following cases (names and other identifying information were modified), taken from Emőke's practice, illustrate the impact of political–historical transgenerational traumas and destructive loyalty and the process of breaking free from these destructive patterns. (Each case's family timeline is marked in Fig. 2.1 in the context of national historical events.)

Case 1. Edit's Story

When she first came to see me, Edit felt she and her family were in constant danger. She was afraid something bad would happen to them. Her cousin had been murdered a short while ago. Her 12-year-old daughter suffered from a serious disease. In exploring her family history, I learned that her great-grandmother had three siblings, and they had lived with their parents on a farm. One of the siblings, István, was a bachelor and lived with the extended family. They were the most affluent farmers in their area. Their possessions—which they acquired with hard work—caused some people to be jealous. When the communists took power in 1948, they brought about violent collectivization, and it reached Edit's family. When the communists arrived in the village looking for an affluent family, István knew the gang was looking for murder so they could set an example. He misled them and said he was the sole owner of the farm so he could save his family. He was dragged away, tortured, and his body was sawed into pieces. He sacrificed himself for his family. Their possessions were collectivized, but their lives were saved.

Decades later, but still during the communist regime, her father took Edit to the house where the brutal crime took place. This had to be done in secret, as the murder was considered an act of setting communist values. It was impossible to fight for justice or to find the ones responsible for the murder. Acknowledging István's act of self-sacrifice, honoring his memory, or expressing gratitude was also not possible, as it would have been against the political system. Edit—just as the other members of the family—listened to the story but tried to keep an emotional distance from this horror. However, the descendants of the family expressed their loyalty toward István, consciously or unconsciously, in various ways.

István's sister (Edit's great-grandmother) had four sons, and they all became police officers, just as one of the grandfather's sons, and Edit's little sister, Évi. None of them pursued a political career in the communist police forces. Their desire was that "this should never happen again." Grandfather died in a motor accident at the age of 46 while on the job as a police officer. (István was also 46 when he sacrificed his life.) At the age of 46, Edit's father became an alcoholic. From Nagy's contextual theory, we may assume that the descendants got into trouble as a result of their "destructive entitlement" (Böszörményi-Nagy, 1984/2013). Her cousin's murder and her daughter's sickness intensified Edit's anxiety, along with the family belief that they do not deserve life; they could get sick, even killed.

The turning point of her therapy happened in our psychodrama group. With the help of this method, Edit experienced an emotional breakthrough. She felt all the suffering, István's soul, her own emotions, and those of her family. What had been impossible for generations happened at last! From the role of István, full of empathy, she could speak out the liberating message: "I did this so that you could live and be happy. I want to see you happy. Suffering belongs to my life only!" At the end of the psychodrama process she said: "I will not pass on this trauma. I am breaking the line." And so it happened. Soon she realized that life was easier. She felt relieved and joyful. Her daughter recovered from her illness and became a successful athlete. After breaking free from the destructive mandate, Edit gained access to the positive resources of her family. Now she is able to pass on humor, vitality, and courage to her family and her social environment.

Related Societal-Level Healing

Recently, Hungarians started to face the past traumas and their effect on the functioning of the family. The House of Terror Museum was opened in 2002. The venue is symbolic: the political secret police of both the Nazis and the communists had their headquarters in the same building where we can now see an exhibition about the victims and the victimizers of the two totalitarian dictatorships. The building also serves as the center for research of the time period (https://www.terrorhaza.hu/en).

Case 2. Kati's Story

I first met Kati when she started dating her husband, Gábor. She had to gain strength to commit to him. In the next phase of the therapy, she processed her mother's death, recognizing the related trauma. After a longer break, she came back a few months pregnant. I assisted her in becoming a mother. Again she needed strong mental support. Alternating periods of supportive and intensive therapy followed. She always asked for help and encouragement when new phases began in her life. Time and time again, she thought she should divorce her husband and stay alone. Interestingly, this idea always came when her relationship with her husband was good. In the last 2 years, we have been processing the political–historical transgenerational trauma in her life.

Great-grandfather was a rich Jewish factory-owner. He lost all his possessions due to the persecution of the Jews and died in poverty. Ilona (grandfather's sister) was taken to a forced labor camp with her husband and two children because of their Jewish origin. They were all killed. Before being taken to labor service, Ilona and her family visited grandfather. Grandmother urged Ilona to leave the children with them; as she was not Jewish, the children would be safe with her. Ilona responded: "Family is the most important. We will stay together." This statement had great significance. In the extended family Ilona was the woman who was able to commit to her husband and dared to have children despite the patterns she had seen. For her, family was of utmost value. But it was exactly the ultimate respect of this value that caused the death of her children during those horrible times.

Grandfather was also taken to labor service because of his Jewish origin. He returned. As the result of all the persecution he suffered as a Jew, he kept his origin a secret from his children as well as the terrible fate of Ilona and her family. None of his children knew about the devastation the Holocaust had caused for their family. However, they carried on the destructive mandate. They were engaged in bitter family inheritance disputes, and this angry state of mind helped them keep a distance from the horrible memories of the Holocaust. Two years ago, Kati found grandfather's diary, which allowed her to discover what had happened to Ilona and her family. It was around the time when her cousin, Sándor, committed suicide due to a psychotic episode. He hallucinated about terrible monsters. As it turned out later, his father, Miklós, and his brother had had similar hallucinations. But just as they never talked about the extermination of Ilona and her family, their paranoid nightmares had not been mentioned either. They kept silent, angry, and busy with their disputes, thus passing on the destructive mandate. They never shared their own experiences.

While reading grandfather's diary, Kati went through a deep crisis. For the first time in her life, she faced what had happened to her family, including the most horrible details. In her dreams, she met the monsters and witnessed the deaths. In this sensitive state, Kati started to feel a strong connection to the 12-year-old Anna, one of the dead children. With the help of the "empty chair technique," we brought Anna into the therapy space. Speaking from the role of Anna, Kati told about the life she planned for herself and the meaning of joy and love she learned from her parents. She had been dreaming about her future, family, and children. After a lot of crying, Anna asked Kati to continue with life where hers had to end. She told Kati to be happy, express her desires, love herself—dare to love her husband and her children, and to live in a family. For Anna, the idea that "family is important" brought about her death, but Kati did not have to tear her family apart in order to save her children.

This encounter filled Kati with strength and motivation. Thanks to Anna's words, the family mandate has changed. Until then, following her destructive mandate, her life was ruled by shame, unhappiness, and guilt. Now it all became a thing of the past. Kati started to experience the joy of standing up for herself and her children. Her children's lives have changed too. Her daughter was taken to a new school community where she is loved and able to soar. The transgenerational effect of the outside destruction, hopefully, ends here.

Related Societal-Level Healing

After decades of silence, the opportunity opened for processing the trauma of the Holocaust. The Holocaust Memorial Center is not only an exhibition; it also conducts a complex activity as a documentation, scientific, and educational center. After past waves of antisemitism, according to the leaders of the Jewish community, the Jewish population enjoys safety in Hungary. There is zero tolerance to antisemitism, and Holocaust denial is prohibited by law (https://hdke.hu/en).

Case 3. Klara's Story

A 49-year-old woman, living with her husband and 5-year-old son, turns to me for help. She felt she is "not good" as a mother, a wife, a daughter, and a sister. She did not feel valuable in her profession as a helper. During the therapy, it turned out that no matter how much she wanted to control herself, she sometimes shouted at her son Peti and even yanked him. She reveals that the same was done to her by her parents, sister, and even her classmates. Though she would have every reason to complain about her parents' conduct, she talks with more passion and pain about the persecutions her parents had to go through.

In 1968, Klara's father wanted to travel to West Germany for his beloved grandmother's funeral. However, he was not granted a passport as he had been to Western Europe within a year. In his disappointment, he wrote a letter to his cousin in West Germany, describing in detail the dictatorship in Hungary. He neglected the fact that letters sent to the West were regularly opened at the border by the authorities, especially when the sender had relatives in Western Europe. Father's letter was opened because the "envelope was damaged." A week later the authorities suddenly came to his workplace. He did not even have a chance to say goodbye to his family; he was remanded immediately. The charge against him was "attempt of public provocation against the People's Republic of Hungary." He was imprisoned for 2 years, his degree in law was withdrawn, and his wife was removed from her job as an administrator. A well-respected notary public until then, at the age of 35 his life, along with the life of his family, changed forever. Their standard of living, as well as their poise, started to decline. Father became an alcoholic, and mother was dissatisfied both with her fate and her husband and became almost completely unsuitable for fulfilling her role as a mother.

Klara was born after father was released from prison. Her strong loyalty as a child enforced the destructive mandate. She lived with the label and shame of having an alcoholic, ex-convict father. At school she was bullied, and the teacher did not protect her, as she was the daughter of that "inmate." She also became the black sheep of the family. Her father loved her the most, but he was also the one who hurt her the most. Just as her parents were hit by the political powers with shame, isolation, and exclusion, she first suffered and later enacted these destructive patterns herself. Guilt, shame, depression, and feeling inferior followed Klara's life. Her parents, both seriously ill, died almost at the same time. Klara was left with the task of looking through their legacy. This meant yet another period of misery for her, as she faced the details of her parents' lives, which cast light on her childhood and her sufferings.

The dysfunctional behavior of her parents had caused Klara much pain and trauma. Now she experienced the same suffering again. She learned more and more details about the political prosecutions and all the lies. She went through deep crises and felt again the anger, suffering, and disappointment that she experienced as a child—all of which were the responsibilities of her parents. Then came the realization: her parents could not have done things differently. They were not guilty, so she could forgive them. She realized that her father was a valuable and loveable man before 1968. If everything had been going on as before, he could have been a good father to her. What followed was the distorted functioning of the victims of dictatorship. Later she could recall those intimate moments when she felt the loving care of her father. She forgave and got rid of the transgenerational burden, and it showed in her relationship with Peti the most. The signs of her dysfunctional parenting disappeared. Their relationship became easier, full of love and humor. She was now able to speak up for her son at kindergarten, clearly and loudly. She decided that she would not let anyone hurt her son any more. She started to use the word "dignity," a concept that was unknown for her family for a long time.

Related Societal-Level Healing

We may acquire information on our predecessors' personal trauma from the Historical Archives of the State Security Organizations. The research of the Historical Archives has been focused on the post-war organization and operation of the political police in Hungary, including the relationship between the Communist Party, the governmental organs, and the public security authorities. The results of this research have been made public in monographs, articles, and selected document publications (https://www.abtl.hu/english-information).

Case 4. Péter's Story

Péter (45) came to see me because he wanted to get rid of his periodic depressive symptoms and alcohol abuse. He wanted to be a good father to his 10-year-old son, Áron, and also wanted to find a woman who could be his partner in life. Áron was two when Péter and his wife divorced. Peter was 2 when *his* parents divorced.

Péter's father was 2 when his father (Péter's grandfather) was drafted to fight in the war and never returned. Péter fought for Áron a lot. His ex-wife denied him all access rights. After many years of dispute with the police and the court, he managed to achieve legally ensured contact with his son. Surprisingly, their relationship remained strong. Péter wants to be a good father. He wants to be able to grant freedom to his son, and let him make friends with children his age. He sees he has work to do concerning his romantic relationships. He is unable to let loved ones close and breaks up instead. Focusing on the past raised a helpful coincidence. All children concerned lost the safety of their families at the age of two, when the fathers disappeared from their lives.

Grandfather was 35 when he was drafted and taken to war in 1943. Until then he had been living with his wife happily. They found joy in their son. But then he had to leave—as it turned out later, to certain death. As most of the wives and mothers left behind, grandmother never learned what had happened to grandfather. All her life, she was unhappily waiting for him to come back, giving up on the pleasures of life. This was the destructive pattern, shaped by external forces, by the destruction of the war, which was passed on to his son Géza, and his grandson, Péter. Grieving the loss of grandfather was hindered by the fact that the official news of his death never arrived. Since these soldiers—approximately 200,000 drafted civilian reservists—fought against the Soviet Union as the allies of Nazi Germany, the communist system considered them war criminals. Family members kept their pain for themselves, and excluded even their children from their emotions, to protect them in case it turned out that they were "enemies of the system." Grandmother was unable to express her emotions, only cried silently in her heart, and repressed her desire for intimacy. Péter's father was unable to open up either to his son or his wife. Yet somehow Péter managed to have a relationship with grandmother full of emotions, which taught him he could have emotional connection with others. However, this connection only forwarded the destructive mandate: "Loving someone is dangerous, you can lose the other person. You'd better avoid intimacy altogether!"

During the therapy, Péter first had to learn to accept his feelings and verbalize his needs, pain, shame, and anger. When he and his father came to session together, they showed such deep understanding toward each other, which later served as the basis of trust in their relationship. Together they recalled memories of Grandfather and Grandmother. They managed to go through the grieving process which had long been overdue. They cried together. After this, the nature of the therapy became supportive. When Péter managed to express his feelings toward his father, the road to forgiveness opened. Péter understood that Father could not have lived differently, nor could he have been a better father. Due to this forgiveness, life-changing energies came to the surface, replacing depression with joy, and self-isolation with the ability for intimacy. Péter also recognized that when he found his own life, this improved Áron's quality of life as well. By facing the unprocessed past of his family he worked not only for himself, but also for his son and the future.

Related Societal-Level Healing

Approximately 2 years ago, nearly 700,000 personal documents arrived in Hungary from Russia. This has great significance in researching the past of Hungarian families since the documents include data of those people who were taken prisoners of war during and after World War II or forced into work camps in the Soviet Union. The documents have been translated to Hungarian and made accessible for the general public. These can help reveal the fates of people that the family members had not known or were not allowed to speak about for decades (https://www.memo.ru/en-us/).

Hope and the Collective Memory of Hungarians

In the examples above, individual families found hope and peace of mind through the therapeutic resolution of past injustices. At a societal level, it is helpful to understand the national identity, attitude, and contemporary social and political circumstances of Hungarians and to take a look at the collective memory of the nation. László et al. (Fülöp & László, 2011; László, 2005, 2011) researched the emotions appearing in Hungarian historical storytelling and found that emotional patterns of Hungarians are characterized by fear, hope, enthusiasm, grief, and disappointment. The patterns of collective memory of Hungarian history have been initial victories followed by defeats, which in turn are not followed by victory, redemption, or reparation—as in the case for the Germans, who lost World War II, but due to the Marshall plan and the economic boom that followed, managed to win the peace after the war (László et al., 2002).

The emotional and cognitive organization of the Hungarian national identity is deeply connected to the glorious distant past, whereas the traumas of the twentieth and previous centuries have not been processed on the cognitive or emotional level. So far, research has shown that on the one hand, collective memory divides history into a remote, glorious past and a consequent series of defeats and losses; on the other hand, it represents the revolutions as events starting with celebrated victories, but ending in oppression and submission. This historical path does not provide a good basis for an emotionally stable identity. The emotions typical of the Hungarian national identity (fear, sadness, disappointment, enthusiasm, and hope) gain their true meaning in one another's context; therefore, it is more reasonable to talk about the emotional pattern of the historical career than about individual emotions (László, 2012).

Hope as an emotion may serve as a suitable example. The cognitive content of hope is different for the Hungarians and for the Americans. Hope is important for American and Hungarian national histories; however, in the American narrative, hope is encompassed by emotions such as confidence, optimism, and security (Bellah, 1967; McAdams, 2006). In Hungarian historical narratives, the Hungarians tend to attribute low agency to themselves. Hope matched with low agency and control is a sign of depressive dynamics (Fülöp et al., 2011). This constellation is characterized by low coping capacity and permanent pessimism. The hope of Hungarians reflects a desire for an incidental favorable turn of events following heavy failures, while the hope of Americans shows an image of an optimistic attitude toward life (László, 2012).

As far as the greatest Hungarian collective trauma, the Peace Treaty of Trianon, is concerned, we attempt to process it via reframing; the anniversary of the Trianon Treaty was named the Day of National Coherence in 2010, when a law was passed to declare all Hungarians, regardless of their official citizenship, members of the unified Hungarian nation. This decreases the significance of administrative borders and strengthens the identity and sense of belonging to the nation. Just as reconciliation took place between the French and the Germans, Hungarians are also interested in settling the relationship with the neighboring countries. One positive example was when in 2013, President János Áder apologized in the parliament of Beograd for the war crimes committed by Hungarians against the Serbs in 1942. During the same visit, a Serbian monument was dedicated by the Serbian and Hungarian president together in honor of the Hungarians who were slaughtered by the Serbs in 1944–45. Today, the relationship between Serbia and Hungary is better than ever before. This serves as a positive model, bringing hope for the future (Szerb Magyar, 2014).

Those who witnessed the middle part of the twentieth century are still among us. We have access to information, which can be talked about. We have therapeutic techniques and experience at our disposal. The window for work is open now. We may never know for how long—the covid pandemic and the threat of war "next door" in Ukraine made it obvious that the series of traumas have not ended. Whatever has accumulated so far, now is our time to process, while we still have the chance. Could it be that our concept of hope will be transformed in the end?

References

Bellah, R. (1967). Civil religion in America. *Daedalus, 96*, 1–21.

Boszormenyi-Nagy, I., & Sparks, G. (2013). *Invisible loyalties*. Routledge. (Original work published 1984 by Brunner/Mazel).

CIA. (2022). *The World Factbook*. https://www.cia.gov/the-world-factbook/countries/hungary/

Fülöp, É., & László, J. (2011). Érzelmek a valós csoportközi konfliktusokban: a csoportközi érzelmek történelmi lehorgonyzása. *Magyar Pszichológiai Szemle, 66*(3), 467–485.

Fülöp, É., Péley, B., & László, J. (2011). A történelmi pályához kapcsolódó érzelmek modellje magyar történelmi regényekben. *Pszichológia, 31*(1), 47–67.

Human Development Reports. (2022). *Human development insights*. https://hdr.undp.org/data-center/country-insights#/ranks

KSH. (2013). *2011. évi népszámlálás – országos adatok*. https://www.ksh.hu/docs/hun/xftp/idoszaki/nepsz2011/nepsz_03_00_2011.pdf

KSH. (2020). *A népesség megoszlása alkoholfogyasztási szokások szerint (2009-)*. https://www.ksh.hu/docs/hun/xstadat/xstadat_eves/i_fek007.html

KSH. (2022a). *Halálozások a gyakoribb halálokok és nem szerint*. https://www.ksh.hu/stadat_files/nep/hu/nep0010.html

KSH. (2022b). *Házasságkötések, válások*. https://www.ksh.hu/stadat_files/nep/hu/nep0015.html

KSH. (2022c). *Magyar állampolgárok vándorlásának összefoglaló adatai*. https://www.ksh.hu/stadat_files/nep/hu/nep0030.html

László, J. (2005). A történetek tudománya. Bevezetés a narratív pszichológiába. *Pszichológiai Horizont, 3*, 209–223.

László, J. (2011). Narrative psychology. In D. J. Christie (Ed.), *The encyclopedia of peace psychology* (pp. 687–691). Wiley-Blackwell.

László, J. (2012). *Történelemtörténetek: Bevezetés a narratív szociálpszichológiába*. Akadémiai Kiadó.

László, J., Ehmann, B., & lmre O. (2002). Történelemtörténetek: A történelem szociális reprezentációja és a nemzeti identitás. *Pszichológia, 2002*(2), 147–162.

McAdams, D. P. (2006). *The redemptive self: Stories Americans live by*. Oxford University Press.

Molnár, M. (2001). *A concise history of Hungary*. Cambridge University Press.

Szabó, M. (1983). *Megmaradt Szobotkának*. Magvető.

Szerb Magyar. (2014). *A historical review of the most painful wounds in the joint past of Serbia and Hungary*. https://2010-2014.kormany.hu/download/1/06/41000/SZERB%20MAGYAR%20EN-végleges.pdf

Valuch, T. (2002). *Magyarország társadalomtörténete: A XX. század második felében* (The history of Hungarian society in the second half of the 20th century). Osiris.

World Economic Forum. (2021). *Global gender gap report*. https://www3.weforum.org/docs/WEF_GGGR_2021.pdf

World Health Organization. (2021). *Global health observatory data repository*. https://apps.who.int/gho/data/node.main.MHSUICIDEASDR?lang=en

Chapter 3
Collective Trauma and Retraumatization in Russia: A View from the Inside

Elena V. Miskova

> *Trauma decontextualized in a person over time can look like personality.*
> *Trauma decontextualized in a family over time can look like family traits.*
> *Trauma decontextualized in a people over time can look like culture.*
>
> —*Resmaa Menakem (2017)*

Three years ago, I was working on my Psychology Master's thesis on multigenerational trauma of Stalin's political repressions in Russia (Miskova, 2019). This subject was not new for me; being a History PhD, a sociocultural anthropologist by my first profession, I was familiar with the problems of collective traumatization within the framework of psychological anthropology, which I taught for many years at the Moscow State University. But still a while ago I treated this subject as being more of an "archeological" nature; despite the importance and gravity of the research topics, it seemed that the traumatic event itself was something removed in time and not immediately threatening us. Today everything changed rapidly; Russia's "special military operation" in Ukraine and all things related have made this an urgent and emotionally charged problem. As a family therapist, I encounter this in my current clinical practice. The question that social researchers and clinicians in Russia are facing today is this: How do the new triggers activate, if they do, the old collective traumas, ensuring the recurrent experiencing of the past and the actualization of the

Translated by Kirill Glebov and Tatiana Glebova

E. V. Miskova (✉)
Center of Medical Anthropology, Institute of Ethnology and Anthropology, RAS, Moscow, Russia

T. Glebova, C. Knudson-Martin (eds.), *Sociocultural Trauma and Well-Being in Eastern European Family Therapy*, AFTA SpringerBriefs in Family Therapy,
https://doi.org/10.1007/978-3-031-29995-7_3

old survival strategies? What is in effect being triggered and what is to be done about the collective emotional process that increases the individual psychological burdens?

Historical Background

Russia's modern history abounds in social cataclysms. At the time of the abolition of serfdom (the ownership of lands and people) in tsarist Russia in 1861, 103 thousand landowners owned ten million peasants (Belovinsky, 1975). The consequences of the centuries-old system of oppression affected the lives of generations of Russians. Social mobility was determined by people escaping and resettling in remote corners of the empire and its extensive colonial policies. World War I led to the mobilization of 15 million Russians and the food crisis. All that was among the factors that brought about the era of revolutions that Russia lived through in the first quarter of the twentieth century.

The most far-reaching was the October Revolution of 1917 that brought communists to power. The establishment of the new regime was followed by a bloody civil war that took the lives of, according to various estimates, between 10 and 17 million people, with 2 more million emigrating (Novikova, 2016). The Bolsheviks' industrialization of Russia was accompanied by the massive eradication of peasantry, which amounted to over 80% of Russia's population before the revolution—over two million were deported and resettled in Siberia and the Far East, and around six million died of hunger. Under Stalin, the Soviet state also conducted mass political repressions against the so-called "enemies of the people", which affected all social strata. These repressions peaked in 1937–38 but lasted until Stalin's death in 1953 and led to mass executions, establishment of an extensive system of forced labor camps (GULAG), and mass deportations of certain ethnicities. There is still no reliable final data about the number of victims, but even the available official statistics indicate several million victims.

World War II, which the country entered in 1941, has in the span of 4 years, according to official estimates, taken the lives of approximately 26.6 million Soviet citizens, of which the majority were Russians (Interfax, 2015). The consequences of this demographic catastrophe have still not been overcome—war-related generational and gender gaps are recurring every 25–30 years. According to the latest demographic pyramid (as of January 1, 2020), the number of 20-year-olds in Russia is almost half of the 35-year-olds, with similar gaps for older generations. Such cycles can repeat themselves for many decades and affect the birth rate and aging dynamics in Russia. Therefore, the composition of the workforce is dominated by older generations, those born at the end of the 1960s and beginning of the 1970s and those born in the 1980s (Media Office, the All-Russian Population Census, 2021).

In the second half of the twentieth century, the Soviet people's life was generally calmer, although there were hushed-up social unrests, ecological disasters (of which the most serious one was the explosion at the Chernobyl nuclear power plant), and wars (the USSR had been carrying out the so-called "international mission" in

Afghanistan for 10 years). The last quarter of the twentieth century saw the collapse of the communist regime, which was accompanied by territorial changes and the "shock therapy" of economic transformation. The 1990s are often described by the generation of people who lived through them and those who were children at that time as a shock to the family and a crisis that actualized many old family traumas.

These days, starting on February 24, 2022, Russia is waging war against its neighbor Ukraine, a former constituent republic of the USSR. People's lives are being destroyed on both sides of state boundaries, and collective traumas are further exacerbated.

Manifestations of Trauma on Collective and Individual Levels

Multiple definitions of collective trauma can be summarized as a forced experience by members of a community of any catastrophic events imprinted in the collective consciousness and drastically and irreversibly changing their identity (Alexander, 2003). Norms, values, and people's behavior rules change, and narratives and symbolic constructs that become the new foundations for the construction of the society are formed.

Hübl (2020) summarized the symptoms of collective trauma as historical trauma response, such as manifestations of tribalism and xenophobia—isolationist sentiments in society. We come across collective denial and abundance of the so-called shadow language in mass communication. The war in Afghanistan was called by the Soviet media "the fulfillment of international obligation," and today in Ukraine Russia is ostensibly conducting a "special military operation"; euphemisms replace direct statements, preventing the admission of complex feelings with respect to the ongoing events. We are faced with multiple social polarizations, from intrafamilial to new conflict splits between various groups and parties. We witness the narrowing of social perspectives, when collective consciousness and vision become tunnel-like, as though from inside a besieged fortress. We see the social loyalty to trauma when the collective identity and communities are being built around the real or implied loss (as in Volkan's concept of "chosen trauma," Volkan, 2001).

At the family level, trauma facilitates the increase of domestic violence and tolerance toward it, including disciplining the children. This can be evidenced by Russia's apparent lack of willingness to adopt the law on the prevention of domestic violence stuck in the parliament since 2016, while at the same time speedily adopting the law on the decriminalization of domestic violence in 2017.

Transgenerational Trauma

Intergenerational trauma is the breakdown in the integrity of Self, a systemic interconnectedness of the identities of different levels—familial, social, and intrapsychic (e.g., Danieli, 1998; Danieli et al., 2015). The multigenerational trauma means not only the transmission of the traumatic experience to the second generation of survivors but also a composite effect and a manifestation of trauma in the form of recurrent survival strategies in several generations. The intergenerational transmission means the transmission of unprocessed traumatic experience whose restructuration becomes the task of the second, third, and further generations. The greater the nonverbal component as well as the volume of the concealed part of this experience (secrets), the more life strategies of descendants will be connected to nonconscious convictions, values, and behavioral models that were fitting for the past but are not up to their life tasks of today.

During reflection and working with collective traumas, it is important to take into account the cultural conditionality of multiple losses—the fact that what, how, and why we are going to consider a loss will depend heavily on the cultural context (Hinton & Good, 2016). Most frequently, we talk about a social loss, a loss of a significant other because of death or separation (migration, deportation). However, besides this, there are cultural losses (loss of cultural traditions and values that stems from revolutions, coups, and occupation) and the impossibility of performing the necessary rites, for example, the inability to carry out the burial of the dead and the perished because of mass violence. Russians today are confronted with a multitude of losses, from the loss of consumer goods and services as a result from withdrawal from the Russian market of many Western manufacturers and commercial companies to the loss of social connections due to the continuing emigration of relatives and friends from Russia as well as loss of life and health by servicemen, both volunteers and conscripts, involved in hostilities in Ukraine.

Many of these losses activate the previous experience of various traumas such as survival under the conditions of deficit or emigration. Despite the current exodus from the country being totally unlike the post-revolution "white" emigration at the beginning of the twentieth century or the "dissident" emigration of the late Soviet period of 1970s–80s, we often perceive it as a one-way ticket and a farewell, thus activating prior cultural meanings to process the new situation. In a situation where grieving for these losses is marked as prohibited and "indecent", the chances for retraumatization and the intergenerational trauma increase rapidly. Therefore, the current stress manifests itself in the forms of multigenerational trauma at the same time.

When I was performing a social and demographic analysis in my research of the trauma of Stalin's repressions, I obtained an interesting portrait of those who bear the burden of loyalty to the traumatic past of their families in the form of various survival strategies. Family projections through maintaining the history and traditions of the family fall mostly on the shoulders of women and the only or eldest children in the family. As expert psychologists who work with family histories in their studies told me, the sphere of emotional contact is culturally more allowed for women and the woman must repair something in the family. These days I also discover an active emotional process regarding the current military conflict among my female clients—many are in open grieving while men more often demonstrate rationalizing and denying defenses.

Collective Emotions and Collective Traumatization and Retraumatization

When working with collective trauma, it is important to consider the reality of collective emotions while keeping in mind that these are qualitatively different than individual emotions (Prikhidko, 2009). Of particular importance for understanding collective trauma are emotions based on group belonging that emerge in connection with events or actions in which a person may not necessarily be personally involved. They often transform into an "emotional burden" or a collective responsibility. The infectiousness of collective emotions is higher. Their virulence is caused by the fact that their underlying affect is transmitted and shared with others before a cognitive assessment, aided by their ever-evolving vehicles—various mass media. Peculiarities of collective emotions ensure the stability and resistance of collective traumas to healing because an individual needs to make a lot of effort to take an emotional responsibility for one's own behavior while not drowning in the collective affect.

I have often been asked why the Russian society in which so many people have been repressed has not produced an unambivalent attitude toward the crimes of Stalin's regime. It appears that the answer lies in the peculiarities of collective affect. Collective guilt is related to responsibility for the past events and implies moral and other kinds of compensation to the victims. In Russia's case, too many people across many generations have been affected and compensation of that scale is perceived as impossible. As for the emotion of collective shame, it is connected to damage to self-image and the related values and therefore blocks prosocial behavior.

As my research shows (Miskova, 2019), at the individual level of working with trauma the factors that lower retraumatization in future generations and increase resistance are the emotional openness and the emotional intimacy transmitted, for example, in a family. Emotional openness is a form of social interaction whereby an expression of emotion is mediated by a sensory modality (body or speech) which is perceived as complete, informative, generating a response, and preventing a simulation and a repression of affect (Keltner et al., 2016). Emotional intimacy means the availability of psychological contact and the intention to open up one's inner world on the basis of trust, acceptance, understanding, compassion, and readiness to emotionally support each other (Collins & Feeney, 2004; Kulikov & Pastushik, 2009). Emotional intimacy is a characteristic of different relationships—parent–children, spousal, romantic, friendships, or collegial. It is only possible given safe communication, and at the collective level, it is an effect that is nearly impossible to achieve and, most importantly, requires a lot of acts at public or societal levels to maintain.

As long as an acute stress reaction continues, people have a potential opportunity to process negative emotions, which arise, among other things, in connection with past experience. Psychologists in Russia are now encountering a lot of triggers of ungrieved grief in clients' stories. Collective trauma almost always presupposes the absence of conditions necessary to process one's losses through rituals by delegitimizing these losses as worthy of mourning. As soon as a culture assumes a heroic posture and starts avoiding heavy emotions, trauma's chances for getting processed diminish drastically.

Quite recently, various conditions for the transformation of collective emotions were shaping up in Russia, including, among others, performance arts, for example, a documentary theater. I worked as a psychologist consultant for one of the shows. The project "Tango Morgen, Tango Pli" by the Novosibirsk Academic Youth Theater "Globus" (Bondarenko & Ivanov, n.d.) was about the experience of women who lived through World War II in Siberia. Actresses read aloud the memoirs of their ancestors and testimonies of their life, thus reestablishing their relatives' right to difficult feelings and assessments. Women of that era who worked their fingers to the bone under the slogan "Everything for the Front, everything for the Victory" could not express their anger and fury toward their husband-heroes who returned from the front, despite them often behaving in an asocial and cruel way. They could not mourn for those who disappeared without a trace but also could not express their doubts and resentment toward them; what if he never returned to her but rather returned to another family? They could not complain about the difference in food supplies for the front and for the interior, where families were often hungry while toiling at back-breaking work. These women's emotional lot was numbing, with insensitivity toward children coupled with overprotectiveness to the degree of cruelty. Giving voice to their complicated feelings, the actresses were forming a therapeutic emotional mode for the show's participants and spectators. Unfortunately, today the space for such emotional processing is winding down, and many emotional losses are impossible to reveal again.

At a recent training on working with the inherited burden in the Internal Family Systems (IFS) model (Schwartz, 2021), we asked our colleagues, mostly women, what associations they had with such words as crisis, "special operation", war, and grief? Having analyzed and categorized their responses, we saw a picture that had few differences from the emotional representations of the grand- and great-grandmothers of the female characters of the theater war play or the heirs of Stalin's repressions trauma from my research. Life's emotional background consists of heavy feelings. The female participants are scared by the imbalance of social roles: men are again a weak link, they can be killed, and they need to be protected while the whole burden of earning one's living will predictably land on women's shoulders. The major threats are perceived to be hunger, poverty, and economic hardship, which activates survival behavior through, for example, stocking up on food. The dominant threats are also enmity, commotion, and division. In this situation, women adopt the attitude of passivity and equalizing behavior—put up with it and don't stand out!

Autoethnography of the Actualization of Collective Trauma

Beginning on February 25, 2022, in the course of the first 2–3 months of the "special operation," I had an opportunity to pursue the autoethnography of collective shock and trauma, studying the ways in which my clients' stories at in-person and online sessions resonated with my own feelings as well as professional experience and studies.

Civil War Outside and Inside

The first obvious reaction was often realized and expressed by clients as relational problems: conflict, "civil war" inside themselves, and on the outside.

The entry in my Facebook (FB) account of February 25:

> I am judging by myself. The self-destruction fire alarm system turned on: the parents passed away, the children grew up, I don't owe anybody anything! I can't, I won't lie anymore! From all this I understand what kind of spring has been squeezing inside all these years. How many civil wars are exploding now inside us again. The parts inside: - stay silent! - one can't keep silent! - there - they are my kin! - and here is your kin, too! - there it is also my land! - here it is also your land! - and what about Dad! - and what about the children??? - and what about the people you should be helping?? - and who is going to help me?!

Questions of how to preserve families, how to talk to the parents who have a different opinion about the current events, and how to communicate with friends on the other side of the societal "barricades" as well as relatives and friends on the other side of the state border were tormenting many people. The behavioral pattern that was self-reproducing was to break connections because it was impossible to come to an agreement but dangerous to stay in conflict. It was dangerous to say one's thoughts aloud, impossible to keep one's convictions while allowing for the opposite views of the other one—it would be necessary to keep fighting until victory. At that moment, clients were making a discovery that even in the "fight for peace" their fighting parts were employing very "military" methods. I watched the behavioral styles which I described in connection with Stalin's repressions trauma get actualized anew. As a basis for research, I took the model of a group of scholars under the leadership of Yael Danieli, which studied the reparative styles of the Holocaust victims' descendants and identified four distinct styles (Danieli et al., 2015). In our case, factor analysis did not identify the same styles. Instead, the sample split into two clusters which I conditionally named "nonemotional fighters" and "emotional conformists." These terms do not imply the availability of access to emotions or a complete lack thereof; rather, they reflect the relationship with their expression or tolerance of what could be considered negative emotions. The patterns of these relationships were shaped in families and adopted by the descendants along with the values and attitudes. In the "emotional" cluster, demonstration of feelings through various displays of affection between family members was welcomed; in contrast, the "nonemotional" cluster mostly centered on providing care and the desire to feed while restraining the expression of feelings. However, neither group could be said to have overcome the trauma. Families from both groups were characterized by overprotectiveness, demands to fight injustice, excessively high expectations of children's success, frequent conversations about "politics," and a transmitted distrust of authorities and official sources of information. All that contributed to shaping the descendants' hyper control, difficulties with self-regulation and relaxation, and heightened attachment to and responsibility for the relatives.

My colleague therapists shared with me that when seeing clients they are often confronted with "fighting" styles and attitudes. Many of the traumatic behavioral models and attitudes are related to fear of violence, problems with rational financial behavior, and adequate self-presentation. In relationships, this is manifested in the inability to trust anyone but one's own family ("others are dangerous") and the inability to let the grown-up children go, stay in balanced partner relationships, or ask for help and talk about one's problems—"keep your mouth shut!", "don't wash your dirty linen in public", express and recognize some negative emotions, for example, sadness, and tolerate one's own and others' emotional states. Such people's family experience is characterized by the abundance of emotional expression and intimacy restrictions. The "fighting" stress-coping strategy manifested itself again in the new crisis situation.

"We Will Probably Not See Each Other Again"

The entry in my FB account of March 11 reflects the state many of my clients described due to the emigration challenges, meaning emotional processes which were triggered by sudden losses.

> Today … no, not today. It is already 2.45 am. So, it was last night in my office, at the end of the session, that yesterday's last client with whom we were discussing his decision to urgently emigrate, said when leaving, "We will probably not see each other again". I returned my friend's call who wanted to discuss with me what words to choose to tell her mom that she had terminal stage cancer, and the doctors delivered her sentence. Then I got into my car and discussed with my daughter which store one should go to to buy the rapidly vanishing "Always" pads. And my youngest daughter texted me that she would arrive late at night because she went to see off her English friend who was advised by his lawyer to leave Russia … then I entered the scheduled conference call with the planned group of support and help for colleagues in Ukraine. Then I decided to go to bed, turned on the falling asleep meditation app … 03:05. 03:06. "We will probably not see each other again …"

One of complicated dilemmas that many people in Russia face is whether to emigrate from the country with the political regime whose actions you cannot agree with or stay hoping that the political atmosphere will change. On the popular social platform Telegram, there appeared many channels and groups in which people support each other. One of the research groups called the new wave of emigration from Russia a "shock one," and one of the Telegram channels is called "And we flew away." Nothing was directly or physically threatening many of those who left Russia before the partial mobilization was declared, but the fear of possible repressions for the criticism of the military "special operation" triggered affectively charged images of collective and family history, which served as an impetus for an urgent departure. Here are some testimonies:

> To leave or not to leave is an old question in the family. And now it was as if a scab was ripped off; history is repeating! It became clear, one must run, one gets nauseous - one throws up, one throws up - one gets better. There was a key question: will the basic trust ever form, or will I always wait for them to come after me? Here (in Russia) there are no chances. (Woman, 31)

> I got scared of 1937—blind rage, and then fear. I packed a suitcase and flew to Mexico, and then the USA. (Woman, 50)

> After the 24th it became clear at once—there will be nothing good. I bought groceries. I really share the statement, "I'm a fool and I didn't get anything done!" I was really possessed by a super idea - leave! Escape! although my family had no history of emigration. But it was ringing in my head all the time, "I will be breaking through to the border!" I felt like I did before my departure in the 90s: as if 20 years didn't pass and we were still at the same ground zero only now we are adults. The planning horizon does not extend beyond this evening. I still live day by day." (Woman, 40)

But those who stay while disagreeing with authorities' policies also feel the heavy burden of uncertainty, guilt, and shame. In social networks, the issues of how much those who stay indirectly agree with the regime and act as collaborationists continue to be hotly debated. In the case of those who remain, the experiences and fears of the past are activated to a no smaller, and probably bigger, extent.

> In front of my eyes is the birch tree with a plaque on which together with my grandson we wrote the name of my grandfather who was repressed. We attached it with my grandson recently because only after Perestroika I found out my grandfather's death story. Of course, it is banging inside my head all the time—it is the same again! We must leave! It's killing me that I cannot just take a seat in the street cafe and say loudly to somebody that I am against the war, that the war is bad! But I am not 20! I can't make up my mind. Does staying mean accepting and justifying? Does resisting mean suffering physically? I am afraid. (Woman, 60)

> Staying and reading the news is scary. I know that when you are being beaten you will not be able not to scream, you won't be able to keep your dignity—this is the experience of violence since childhood. (Woman, 50)

"I Am Not Staying Actively"

I titled one of my written reflections in FB on March 16 with a generalized emotion of my clients shared by me—*I am not staying actively, I am staying passively.* It reflects the feeling of guilt and inferiority that those who remain are prescribed to experience. And already on May 5, I asked myself a question about how many Soviet people lived and preserved themselves in internal emigration:

> I thought about the generations of those who lived in the Soviet Orwellian world, did not fight openly but also did not conform? About my father. How, how did they achieve this??? I don't know. The concept of internal emigration suddenly turned from theory into experience which must be mastered and practiced… Communication will be very selective. On the one hand, it will really polish its quality. We will need to think what and how we will talk about. It's an art form. But, but … It's an isolation regardless of whether you went away or stayed inside a narrow circle. And I understand how eventually people would rise from these trenches into an open attack ending in disaster. Because it is very difficult. And dangerous. You are being undermined from the inside anyway ….

My Internal Cassandra or Reminiscing About the Past

Trying to facilitate the internal dialogue—my own and the clients'—I wrote on March 22 about a part of me which I named my internal Cassandra and which responds to the clients' stories about their own experience.

> I have this part, too. Like many others. Like those who read the "cases" of grand- and great-grandfathers. Like those who knew the life of their grand- and great-grandmothers. Like those who heard stories about the many deprivations that Motherland is so rich with. This part is now screaming, "What don't you understand? What, you don't know what will come next? - You won't be able to breathe, think and speak!!!" And then this part colors this spring reality in hues of panic horror. If I ask it what it wants for me, it will most likely reply "safety", but will say it concisely: run, fool, run! Its concern is that I don't freeze, that I move, and it is using anxiety and fear to save me from paralyzing irrational horror. Being afraid of arrest and torture is rational. At least we have an understanding that this is possible. Our ancestors who lived through this did not have this knowledge when they had to face it. My Cassandra is alert: if she must make me move using panic and reminisce about the future, so be it.

Get Up and Go!

The entry in my FB account of April 1:

> We all carry our inherited burden (our trauma)—it has a lot in common but in every one of us this common part is packed carefully and individually. I notice now how angry I am at many men, even in my therapist's office. Women come mostly full of emotions, grieving, and reflection. Men, however, are often in denial or in a heroic posture … I asked my militant part, what makes it so angry? And it turned out that there is another part, standing perfectly still with bags under her eyes from fatigue and getting ready to put something else on her shoulders. "They will now be getting killed or wounded, they will be disappearing without a trace," says she about the men, "they will be returning without arms or legs, they will start drinking down their bitter lot. They will fight and scream. And you will still have to pray to them because they are the heroes!"

Gender double standard is when there emerges a conflict between the prescribed behavioral scenarios and life attitudes and real-life strategies. This is a legacy of military traumas of different eras in our country and their companion of ungrieved grief or pathological grieving. Women solemnly put men on the pedestal of the "strong man" while taking upon themselves a lion's share of responsibility for many everyday matters and life decisions. These were forced and functioning strategies in situations when the country was suffering huge losses of men's lives while women ensured the survival of the families. These survivalist strategies got easily actualized at different stages of Russia's modern history. For example, many of my 30 to 40-year-old clients bear the trauma of the family split and a radical transformation of family roles and hierarchies in the post-Perestroika period of country's life, especially in the 1990s. It was masculinity that suffered the greatest loss: the men turned out to be unable to feed and support their families and maintain the "strong man" status. They required more time to adapt than women for whom the old patterns came alive—there is no time to grieve and whine, one must do something! It is the children who inherited the losses that were again ungrieved and devalued.

Reflecting on the roots of the gender double standard helps clients to externalize their behavioral patterns and thus strip them of involuntariness. When working within the framework of the IFS model, I offered to my clients to conduct the inventory and the differentiation of their parts, which bear the burdens of the ungrieved grief from various periods, mostly the inherited ones, and do not dare to claim the importance of the current losses.

Maria's Case: "Sort It Out to Put Oneself Together" (Published with Client's Permission)

One of such part inventories was performed when working with my client Maria. This case with a representative of Generation Z illustrates the inherited burden of ungrieved grief, which triggers the trauma several generations away from the initial traumatic event. Maria is 21, and by the time the "special military operation" started she has already been in therapy for 2 years. Her initial request for working with me was caused by difficulties in building relationships with parents, peers, and studies. Maria is a well- educated young woman with a sharp intellect. After finishing school she easily gained admission to several universities, but she could not handle the emotional stress of the very first exam session and dropped out from two colleges. Her demands of herself were excessive due to her family's great expectations.

Maria's parents are from a family of Russian Germans; they maintain relationships with their extended families. Maria's mother and sister teach at one of Moscow's prestigious higher learning institutions. Her father is a journalist. Her family history includes difficult times of her grandmothers' life in territories occupied by the Nazis during World War II. The family's internal boundaries are blurred: togetherness and loyalty to the family come above everything else. Family members' right to make mistakes is not recognized. Internal anxiety and pressure are constantly intensified by a large volume of shame: "We are different, we are alien and therefore we stand out, we are noticeable. We must be twice better and more responsible than everybody else to resist the condemnation and prevent it". For a while in the 2000s the family lived in Germany where Maria's father had a job. Upon return to Russia, family members encountered constant judgment by society; for example, Maria's elder sister was teased by other children at school who called her "Hitler."

During therapy with the IFS model, Maria spent a lot of time getting to know parts of her personality and unloading parts filled with the burden of perfectionism, shame, and being different, which were reflected in her external relationships: she got admitted to a university and successfully finished her first year of studies, formed a circle of friends, found a first job, and started to build dyadic relations with her mother, father, and sister. She not only changed her life, but also learned to own her achievements as well as treat herself with compassion, allowing for the necessity and inevitability of mistakes.

However, after February 24—the beginning of war with Ukraine—Maria showed regression in her emotional condition but was able to differentiate her parts, take a self-observation stance, and reflect on self-regulation failures. During one of our sessions she told me that she "lost herself":

> Everything is objectively not bad— I love my college, I got a job, communication got going, I built a relationship with my parents. But I always have a feeling that I won't be able to finish something, that everything can be taken away from me or that I will change so much that I won't need anything anymore.

Maria explained what provoked the anxiety:

> Dad came home from work gray faced. The euro crashed, and he is getting his salary in euros, and his organization can be declared a foreign agent any day now, and he might get fired. He emptied his pockets. This sound of small change on the table! I found myself in one of my childhood moments: 1990s, a family trip to the park, an underground crossing, the paupers asking for alms, somebody's playing a guitar. Mom, sarcastically," Oh, you can do it with your Dad—you'll sing, he'll collect the money". Shame and fear. Dad is bitter but keeps silent. The family at that time was repeating like a mantra, "We are not going to buy anything, we don't have the money", but at the same time you must be the smartest ones, the most interesting ones so that nobody would ever call your sister a Hitler in school again. I remember and I feel that fear: Dad will not be able to cope! It turns out that Dad - my beautiful, smartest Dad is not all-powerful! Something must be done!

Maria had a mixed feeling of being ashamed and hurt for her father who himself was carrying grandmother's shame for her wartime life under the German Nazis and the impossibility of expressing the grief which their family felt then along with other families. Since then, all of her criticism was directed toward her mother, seemingly more powerful and capable of handling more, while her father became the object of close attention and care. The contact with him became an obsession. Maria was collecting her father's stories. Being in a parentified position, she felt the need to carry the emotions that her father was incapable of expressing. In the present, this necessity was actualized but was now perceived as an anxiety-generating internal polarization:

> If I forget (my family's and my dad's history), it would be as if I became someone shallow, someone bad, a traitor! But if I keep on remembering it, I will lose my mind! I sense behind all this, behind the back the enormity, the huge deposits of grief, but nobody cried! These parts are afraid: if they don't pull apart, the dam will break, and I will not be able to swim out of these tears.

After studying the goals and the tasks of this polarization as well as the exiled (dissociated) parts, we managed to take the inherited burden off Maria's internal system. She began to visualize grief as things packed into suitcases and a memory as an archive which you can use, take something out, and describe it, but not as a dangerous element that can break through the internal dam at any moment and requires enormous efforts to restrain it. The process was also aided by the grieving for Maria's current losses: for example, the legalization of anger and sadness over the loss of possibility to use the customary hygienic products produced a releasing effect. I was grateful to my client and my own daughters for making such losses visible and meaningful for me: the "goodbye to McDonald's" party that my children organized became one of the most important stages of recognizing the transformations happening to us and the accompanying grief.

Conclusion: War Is a Family Album

It seems appropriate to conclude this autoethnographic essay with my FB entry on April 5:

> A young man, who grew up on Chechen wars—literally, he was growing up at that time, told me yesterday, and, with his permission, I will quote: "I am watching the films from Bucha like a family album. It is I who is again walking between the corpses in the streets. And two contradictory and useless feelings pursue me: guilt—although what am I guilty of? and cold-blooded gloating—do you Russians understand now what it is like, although what does it have to do with anything, and what all those who have never been to war can know or understand about the people lying around in Ukrainian streets?"
>
> And a woman from a Siberian city told me, "I keep hearing this voice that sounded in my head when I read the news on Feb. 24, "Russia cannot be an aggressor, we cannot attack! We can't!" And behind that voice and image: My Dad, 13 years old, is turning shells for the front all day long at an evacuated factory during World War II to fight the Nazis …"
> If only we could remember this: any war anywhere on Earth is our common family album!

During the moments of acute social crises and collective traumatization, the weak links of individual adaptive strategies become clearly visible. As the Russian saying goes, "it's where it's thin that it rips apart" (a rough equivalent of "a chain is only as strong as its weakest link"). The anxiety and the emotional flooding uncover what people managed to cope with some time ago, but at a very steep price—that of emotional withdrawal and cognitive distortion. The pillars that were internalized without reflecting, out of loyalty to family values and convictions, become fragile (e.g., Danieli et al., 2015; Levin, 1997).

When the internal harmony of experience and levels of functioning is ruptured, and the pillars fall out we should study the values and convictions that supported them. The study of the intergenerational transmission of the traumatic family experience is especially useful in the current crisis to prevent the "reminiscing about the future" (trauma processing) from providing us with habitual defenses. I think that in such cases we can use trauma healing approaches aimed at the lowering of anxiety and stress in the internal system by decreasing the rigidity of multigenerational defense strategies.

The main task is to ensure that the wheel of the trauma does not turn again at the point when social triggers actualize the habitual emotional reaction and old survival strategies. At such moments it is important to (1) allow for the individual and collective acknowledgement of the losses and grieving over them; (2) leave open the opportunities for exploring and discussing histories on different levels—from individual and family to community; (3) look for the ways to cope with the crisis based on the current evaluation of the situation, available resources, and options; and (4) create images of the future and build plans for what lies ahead based on realizing one's own values and reactivating them in the process.

References

Alexander, J. (2003). *Meanings of social life: Cultural sociology*. Oxford University Press.

Belovinsky, L. V. (1975). Landlords. In *Great Soviet Encyclopedia* (3rd Ed., 1969–1986). Soviet Encyclopedia. http://niv.ru/doc/encyclopedia/bse/articles/13463/pomeschiki.htm

Bondarenko, E. & Ivanov, A. (n.d.) Tango morgen, Tango pli. Novosibirsk Academic Youth Theater "Globus". https://www.globus-nsk.ru/spektakli/tango-morgen-tango-pli/

Collins, N. L., & Feeney, B. C. (2004). An attachment theory perspective in closeness and intimacy. In D. J. Mashek & A. Aron (Eds.), *Handbook of closeness and intimacy* (pp. 163–189). Psychology Press.

Danieli, Y. (1998). Introduction: History and conceptual foundations. In Y. Danieli (Ed.), *International handbook of multigenerational legacies of trauma* (pp. 1–21). Plenum Press.

Danieli, Y., Norris, F. H., Lindert, J., & Paisner, V. (2015). The Danieli inventory of multigenerational legacies of trauma, Part I: Survivors' posttrauma adaptational styles in their children's eyes. *Journal of Psychiatric Research, 68*, 167–175. https://doi.org/10.1016/j.jpsychires.2015.06.011

Hinton, D. E., & Good, B. J. (2016). The culturally sensitive assessment of trauma: Eleven analytic perspectives, a typology of errors, and the Multiplex Models of Distress generation. In D. E. Hinton & B. J. Good (Eds.), *Culture and PTSD: Trauma in global and historicalperspective* (pp. 50–114). University of Pennsylvania Press.

Hübl, T. (2020). *Healing collective trauma*. Sounds True.

Interfax. (2015, November 13). *The Ministry of Defense clarified the losses of the USSR in the Great Patriotic War*. Interfax.ru. https://www.interfax.ru/russia/479070

Keltner, D., Tracy, J., Sauter, D. A., Cordaro, D. C., & McNeil, G. (2016). Expression of emotion. In L. Feldman Barett, M. Lewis, & J. M. Haviland Jones (Eds.), *Handbook of emotions* (4th ed., pp. 467–482).

Kulikov, L. V., & Pastushik, M. M. (2009). Review of foreign studies on the problem of emotional intimacy, Bulletin of St. Petersburg University. *Sociology, 12*(4), 161–167.

Levin, P. (1997). *Waking the tiger: Healing trauma*. from English. North Atlantic Books.

Media Office, the All-Russian Population Census. (2021, June 22). *How the echo of the war affected the young generation of Russians*. https://www.strana2020.ru/mediaoffice/kak-ekho-voyny-otrazilos-na-molodom-pokolenii-rossiyan/

Menakem, R. (2017). *My Grandmother's hands: Racialized trauma and the pathway to mending our hearts and bodies*. Central Recovery Press.

Miskova, E. V. (2019). The trauma of stalinist repression in the context of collective trauma of genocides. *Psychology and Psychotherapy of the Family, 4*, 31–49. https://doi.org/10.24411/2587-6783-2019-10005. https://cyberleninka.ru/article/n/travma-stalinskih-repressiy-v-kontekste-kollektivnyh-travm-genotsidov/viewer

Novikova, L. G. (2016). Civil war 1917–22. In *Big Russian encyclopedia*. https://bigenc.ru/military_science/text/2375223.

Prikhidko, A. (2009). Emotional socialization: Content and mechanisms. *Psychological Studies, 2*(6), 1–15. https://doi.org/10.54359/ps.v2i6.974

Schwartz, R. C. (2021). *No bad parts: Healing trauma and restoring wholeness with the internal family systems model*. Sounds True.

Volkan, V. D. (2001). Transgenerational transmissions and chosen traumas: An aspect of large-group identity. *Group Analysis, 34*(1), 79–97. https://doi.org/10.1177/05333160122077730

Chapter 4
Identity, Security, and Belonging: Healing from Sociocultural Trauma in Romania

Gáspár György

I started working on this chapter on the last days of one of the most rabid Februarys in decades. On the 24th of February, we celebrate Dragobete—which is the Romanian version of Valentine's Day. But, in 2022, this day marked an extremely painful historic moment for the entire planet. Around 5 a.m., the alarms on our smartphones started beeping to let us know that the president of Russia, Vladimir Putin, declared war on our neighboring country, Ukraine. Between Romania and Ukraine, there is a 650-km border, which means that a good part of the north of our country is very close to the country currently at war. The national news showed overwhelming images of bombed buildings and Ukrainians that slept by hundreds in the subways; we hear unbearably sad stories about children who are leaving their fathers behind to follow their mothers in the refugees' convoys that chose to come to or just transit Romania. Our hope is cultivated by the hundreds of Russians that protest against the war and who are willing to take unimaginable risks.

I spent all day Thursday, the 24th of February—from 9:00 in the morning until 20:00 in the evening—at my psychotherapy practice, where I work with adults, couples, and families to help them navigate the complexities of modern relationships. This has been my work for more than 16 years. On that day, most of my psychotherapeutic conversations started with the theme of war. Some clients talked about how they contacted their relatives in the West and central parts of Europe to make sure they have a place of refuge should they need one. Others asked me how they should approach the subject of war with their children so that they wouldn't convey worry, but not deny reality. At the same time, there were some clients who, between tears, told me that they knew what war meant, and that they could not understand how it was possible for a third world war to start when we barely escaped the biological war with the Covid-19 virus.

G. György (✉)
Multicultural Association of Psychology and Psychotherapy, Bucharest, Romania

T. Glebova, C. Knudson-Martin (eds.), *Sociocultural Trauma and Well-Being in Eastern European Family Therapy*, AFTA SpringerBriefs in Family Therapy,
https://doi.org/10.1007/978-3-031-29995-7_4

My clinical and psychotherapeutic work occupies a significant part of what life means to me. From the beginning of 2000 when I discovered family therapy and the psychology of relationships, I felt new doors toward the future have opened for me and that, finally, I hold the necessary instruments to do something for the Romanian people. The systemic way of thinking, which defines the vision of family therapists, represented the exact paradigm I needed to understand both the dynamic and torment of our sociocultural context. It was then that I committed to myself to bring collective trauma to the surface because we cannot mourn what we don't allow ourselves to feel. To move forward, we need to be able to get out of the rusty chains of the past and settle our accounts with our psychological and cultural history; we need to find the words to express the pain and to feel all the experiences that we have frozen inside ourselves. And yes, we can say we survived, but the unhealed past will still burden us until we make peace with it. My mission and the mission of my fellow colleagues from the Association of Multicultural Psychology and Psychotherapy is to reveal what is inside our culture, because what lies inside can be our salvation; but if we are not able to reveal what is inside, it will destroy us.

Romania—A Place Filled with History in the Heart of Central Europe

Romania is the 12th largest country in Europe and is surrounded by Bulgaria, Ukraine, Hungary, Serbia, Moldova, and the Black Sea (see Map A.4, Appendix, this volume). Nevertheless, in the world, we are largely known as the country situated in the southeast part of Central Europe, famously known for the mystical stories about Transylvania and the unmet beauty of the Carpathian Mountains. We may get offended when the capital of our country, Bucharest, gets mixed up with Budapest, the capital of Hungary (which happens more often than you would think), and we like to pride ourselves on the fact that we lived on this land since prehistoric times when our country was called Dacia. At the present moment, Romania has a territory of 238,397 km and a population of approximately19.19 million inhabitants, of which 88.92% are Romanian, 6.50% are Hungarian, 3.29% are Romany, and 1.29% are of other ethnicities (Ukrainians, German, Turkish, Hun, Russian, Serb, Slovak). More than 92.5% of the people are Christian (81% orthodox, 6.2% protestant, 5.1% catholic), and the rest of the 7% declare themselves as having no religion or having non-Christian beliefs. Life expectancy is 71.4 years for men and 78.8 years for women. The divorce rate is increasing significantly: in 2019, one of four marriages ended in divorce; the pandemic exacerbated this phenomenon—we presently register one divorce in every 3.5 marriages (Institutul Naţional de Statistică, 2022).

The Psychological Inheritance of the Communist Regime

Until 1989, Romania was a communist country, and the Romanian people were dominated for decades by the communists with dictator Nicolae Ceauşescu as their symbol. His atrocities induced deep collective trauma for generations of Romanians. Following the suffering imposed by the two world wars, Romanians had to endure their freedoms and democratic rights brutally confiscated; Romanians had to accept new rules imposed on them by the Soviet Union. In the second part of 1944, Soviet troops occupied Romania and implemented a political regime with no social classes and no private property, inducing the idea that the whole country would belong to the big mass of Romanian workers.

For 17 years, from 1947 to 1964, Romania seemed like a national prison. Once the Security (Department of State Security) was set up in 1948 (just a few months after the abdication of King Mihai in December of 1947), the intellectuals and former political people were thrown into penitentiaries, where most of them lost their lives. Starvation, torture, and forced labor were life's routine for those who dared oppose the regime or talk badly about communism. Officers, priests, students, peasants, and even high school students were awakened by Security people and put inside those criminal prisons, thus losing their freedom, family, and even life. The Security became so powerful that their officers had the right to shoot anyone on the spot with no restriction or trial. Some Romanians were considered "enemies of the people" and nationalization of resources began to unfold, through which absolutely everything would become the property of the state. Romanians no longer owned restaurants, stores, hotels, or factories, and not even cars. Many were thrown out of their own homes, which became the houses of communist leaders.

After these years of maximum terror and psychological and emotional insecurity, in 1964, the communist leader Gheorghe Gheorghiu-Dej freed the political prisoners and announced a regime change. A year later, after his death in March, the ambitious and determined Nicolae Ceauşescu took over leadership of the Romanian Communist Party, becoming General Secretary and then Chief of State in 1967.

In the first few years, Romanians had a good impression of Ceauşescu, who liked to be addressed as "beloved leader." He continued the emancipation and liberation politics of the former leader, giving hope again to the Romanian population. The country started to reopen communication channels with the outside world, and science, culture, and art started to flourish again. From 1964 to 1971, the standard of living grew significantly: grocery stores were full again, you could buy magazines in French, you could own a car, dress better, listen to modern music, and alongside Dacia (the car factory), Pepsi-Cola opened its first factory in Romania—the only one in the whole communist territories. It all seemed like something out of a movie, and for a while Romanians managed to cover their traumas with all sorts of rituals and habits, thinking that the worst was in the past. Not only the Romanian people but also their "beloved leader" hid some trauma and psychological unprocessed wounds that, after 1971, were to become visible due to his cruelty and the strictness of his behavior. From a psycho-traumatological point of view, his cruelty could be explained by an abusive childhood and various emotional wounds.

Nicolae and his wife, Elena, went on to become the national symbol of Romania. Slowly, Ceauşescu's image was present in all school materials, on the walls of public institutions, and even in the House of the People. Possibly to compensate for a tormented childhood, Nicolae asked all the stadiums and big boulevards in all the large cities in Romania to acclaim him every time their beloved comrade passed by. Students became Falcons of the Nation and pioneers who, like extras in a movie, rehearsed for weeks on end so that the tribute to the beloved leader would meet his expectations. And even if we had no political prisoners, all those who opposed or criticized the regime were to be declared mentally ill and isolated in mental hospitals. The informants multiplied like mushrooms after a rainy day—you never knew who would turn you into the hands of the Security—so trusting anyone became a real danger. Microphones hidden in people's homes, among other coercive measures, made it so that anxiety turned to obsession and neighbors, relatives, and colleagues were seen with a maximum of suspicion and mistrust.

Historians tell us that life was still bearable until the beginning of the 1980s when Ceauşescu decided to erase Romania's external debt, a debt he made while building heavy industry factories that turned out to be big consumers of energy and highly inefficient from an economical viewpoint. Austerity measures—impossible to imagine in the modern world—were imposed so that everything produced in our country could be exported and the population made to barely survive—perhaps similar to how the family of the child Nicolae Ceauşescu used to live. In the almost empty stores, the only things you could find were jars of vegetable stew, all other aliments were rationed. I still remember the ration books we used during my childhood—we would get 1 kg of sugar and one of meat, 1 L of oil, some butter, and a few eggs that had to be enough to feed a family for an entire month. Fuel was also rationed. And when you were allowed to use the car, you had to make do with the 20 liters of gasoline available per month. All sorts of sweets, citrus fruits, and also razor blades, underwear, and toilet paper were luxury products.

When we went to the outhouse of my grandparents in the countryside, we used newspapers instead of toilet paper, but this was not unusual in the city either. We only had access to hot water twice a week for 2 hours and on the weekend. To take a bath, all the family members used to bathe in the same water so that no one would end up unwashed. The radiators were more cold than hot and housewives cooked at night because the pressure of the gas stove was bigger then. The electricity used to go out a lot and you could never tell how long you would have to stay in the dark or when you would be able to do things around the house. Starting in 1985, the only television station in Romania would transmit 2 hours every night and a few more hours during weekends; the program consisted of infinite honors for the comrades Nicolae and Elena Ceauşescu. All of this ended in December 1989. Though the communist dictatorship in Romania ended that winter, the trauma it caused still haunts the people of the "beloved leader."

If we consider the way Romanians regard themselves, their relationships, and the world, the psychosocial profile is dominated by a lack of self-confidence or trust in others (David, 2015). The lack of openness toward healing their trauma and diminished emotional and relational intelligence make us generally less cooperative and understanding, even in terms of mutual benefits. Prof. Daniel David (2015), rector of the Babeş-Bolyai University (one of the most important Universities in Romania), concluded that lack of cooperation is the main obstacle that stays in the way of Romanians expressing their intelligence and creativity, and this leads to performing below our level. The results of this phenomenon are mirrored by ambivalence and incongruence—an exaggeration of the positive on the one hand, together with negativity and mistrust on the other. According to Prof. David, this social profile is born out of collective chronic uncertainty and unsafety through a long history.

Understanding Trauma and Our Relational Selves

According to Peter Levine (2010), trauma isn't held in the external event that induces physical or emotional pain because trauma is not the event itself but our body's response to what happens to us in the absence of an empathetic witness. Trauma is born when we are not capable of freeing the energy that gets stuck in the body, which would enable overcoming our emotional and physiological responses to painful experiences. If we carefully look at how the Romanian people tend to function, we will discover that we still have entire generations paralyzed by fear who would do anything to avoid confronting their inner demons.

In the book *Psychology of the Romanian People*, Professor David (2015) stated that Romanians tend to present a defensive psychological profile, defined by suppression, the denial of negative aspects, and the tendency to do anything humanly possible to reduce the negative aspects, together with a tendency to amplify the positive ones. Despite these mechanisms, the reactions of the Romanian people are often manifested through behaviors of rejection, violation, and infringing of rules. Our self-esteem can be thought of in three main categories: low self-esteem, compensated self-esteem, and healthy positive self-esteem. Often, you can sense the ghost of Ceauşescu in a superiority complex that suggests compensated self-esteem that mirrors the tendency some of us have in talking of excellence, e.g., the wonderful Olympians of the country and our exceptional performances—when the reality is quite different, because the Olympians are a minority not representative of our educational and professional systems in general.

The relational paradigm posits that our "Self" is deeply relational and that healthy development is possible in a secure and nurturing interpersonal space. From this perspective, the above explanations can be understood as follows: if our need for a secure connection is not met, our Self gets distorted and searches for ways to develop the best it can. Trauma is not the negative experience per se (war, violence, oppression, famine, tyranny, etc.), but the effect that all these atrocities have on the connection with the self, others, and the world we live in (Maté, 2004, 2021; Levine, 2010, 2022).

David (2015) stated that Romanians have a lower level of happiness and life and work satisfaction compared with other European nations or the USA. Unlike the Americans, Romanians have higher scores for features such as amorality, misanthropy, antisocial attitudes, controlled hostility, cynicism, disregard, and masculinity.

Bassel van der Kolk (2015) suggested that trauma also has the power to create changes in the central nervous system, which can alter how we remember things and leave us reactive to stimuli that unconsciously mirror our original experiences. We can thus understand why Romanian women have huge difficulties with shame and anxiety, and Romanian men score high when it comes to generalized fear, competition, and repression (David, 2015). When a family or community system fails to offer traumatized people validation and the empathic witness that could offer a degree of safety, resilience cannot express itself and all that is left is baggage of post-traumatic stress symptoms (Levine, 2022).

The Romanian people, like many others around the world, have suffered from the lack of empathy and humanity of the communist regime. But the real problem is represented by the fact that the majority of us don't dare, not even today, to talk about the terror and the panic that were once a usual part of our day-to-day life. Partly from a lack of education, partly to feel less vulnerable, our great-grandparents, our grandparents, and our parents consciously or unconsciously decided not to break the silence and to move through life as if the past is of no importance. But as Heinrich Pestalozzi said, "You can banish the devil from your garden, but you will find it in the garden of your son" (Miller, 2019, p. 33).

The aftermath of trauma and post-traumatic stress manifests through disruptive emotional states, unwanted behaviors, irrational beliefs, sleep disorders, eating disorders, addiction, and an infinite number of relational problems that worsen anxiety disorders, depressive manifestations, irritability, and uneasiness, hostility, self-harming behaviors, lack of interest in pleasant or ritualistic activities, emotional disconnection, and avoidance strategies and social isolation (Eger, 2021; Levine, 2022; Siegel, 2018).

Exposure of generations of Romanians to the chronic stress induced by the two world wars and then by the atrocities of the communist regime shows up in my clinical practice, and the work of my colleagues around the country, in the following areas of Romanian functioning:

- Connection, human attachment, and trust in others—when babies cannot experience connection with their attachment figures who are paralyzed by fear, drained by terror, and lack of food, the child's capacity for attachment is wounded and can be later noticed in the future relationships, romantic and parental. Thus, Romanian trauma travels through time.
- Neurobiological development and emotional regulation—the mind, relationships, and biological body are indisputably connected. Trauma is not only visible through how we connect with others but also through our emotional and biological development. Often, traumatized children end up developing a low tolerance to stress and have major difficulties in managing emotions and may have an

altered level of language development, abstract thinking, planning, and the capacity to learn from lived experiences.

- Dissociation, denial, and the downplay of pain—as we said before, Romanians are the masters of these mechanisms. Many of today's adults live with the societal narrative that the abuses they experienced during childhood were good for them because being beaten was "a thing from heaven," and that the only reason they succeed in life is due to their parents' toughness and severity. Dissociation, as a natural reaction to trauma, contributes to a low degree of self-awareness, living more in their minds and denying the reactions of their bodies. When not aware of our traumas and/or hiding behind denial when we face the various challenges of life, instead of being guided by the question *What can we do now?,* we may let ourselves be crushed by the question *Why us?*

As a relational psychotherapist, I am especially focused on the effect of trauma on interpersonal functioning. Under the impact of trauma, relationships become altered and distorted because people's capacity for connection, trust, and reciprocity is wounded (Hübl, 2020). And when our relational safety is nonexistent, we have less resilience and more fragility in the face of negative experiences, even losing our sense of self-stability. Even though the communist regime fell more than three decades ago, our great-grandparents', grandparents', and parents' trauma is still alive in us.

The interpersonal relationship profile of the Romanian people (David, 2015) suggests a more anxious-insecure attachment style than in other European states (France, Germany, Lithuania, Portugal, Greece) or in the USA. At a declarative level, we may tend to express an increased desire for a secure attachment style. When we talk about friendship, we are not as open as the Americans, considering the family as more important. With the few friends we have, we tend to get more emotionally involved. My clinical experience shows that, sometimes, we Romanians tend to be almost symbiotic and fusional. This phenomenon is easily explained by the fact that during the communist regime and the Security, whoever saw things "differently" was considered an enemy of the system and thus differentiation and individuation were seen as dangerous.

Healing the Romanian Mental System

Living with the intergenerational effects of a totalitarian system that makes interpersonal connections unsafe and untrustworthy, while also necessary to survival, is often reflected in an ambivalent attitude about life and relationships. This is an indicator of trauma, which in time, distorts the way we see reality, obstructing our views of the world and its opportunities. Siegel (2003) described trauma as an expressive mixture of behaviors that indicate a cognitive rigidity and a state of emotional chaos, aspects that are readily identified in the Romanian people. The healing process, the psychotherapeutic framework, and especially the client–psychotherapist relationship must thus represent a reliable relational experience that, over time, helps one move toward a coherent image of self integrated across body, mind, and relationships (Siegel, 2012). Just as every one of us, regardless of age, culture, education, or gender identity, is unique, so is the psychotherapeutic process co-created between the client and the therapist. The secret lies in clinicians' capacity to understand and hold the subjective experiences of the person(s) they are working with, a process that contributes substantially to the psychological reorganization of the self.

In terms of intimate and family relationships, the goal is to develop the capacity to be open to the experience of another, an integration of minds (Siegel, 2012). Integrated development of the child and the capacity to be aware of and regulate emotion is greatly dependent on the capacity of the parent or the caregiver to show attention and empathy toward the subjective experience of the little one. Studies show that those parents who are more coherent in the realm of inner subjectivity or who can find meaning in their existence have a major positive impact on the development of a secure attachment in their children (Siegel, 2012). Thus, the subjective state and the interpersonal state are intertwined and contribute significantly to what we call well-being (which is the opposite of trauma).

In *Healing Trauma*, edited by Marion F. Solomon and Daniel Siegel (2003), Siegel identified 13 basic elements for the healing process to unfold: connection, compassion, contiguousness, cohesion, consistency, continuity, clarity, co-construction, complexity, consciousness, creativity, and community. Each of these aspects is relevant to my clinical practice in general, and especially when it comes to sociocultural trauma intervention or its manifestation in someone's life.

A Case Illustration

Maria is a client whose life story fits the theoretical framework of the ideas presented in this chapter. Maria is a pseudonym used to protect client identity, but who gave me her consent to present a short version of her life story in this chapter. Born into a family with five children, Maria grew up in an environment that lacked proper affection, and she was hyper-responsible for the well-being of her younger siblings. Maria's parents were little during the Second World War and, broadly, their youth was marked by the burden of the communist regime. In one of our therapy sessions, Maria told me how disconnected she always felt from her parents and how she yearned all her life to gain their appreciation and validation. The reason she reached out to me as a therapist was due to some states of anxiety and uneasiness that were burdening her life and distracted her from what she wanted to do.

Following the clinical model of interpersonal neurobiology (Siegel, 2003), the main objective (with each client) is that of building a therapeutic relationship, to create a *connection* that could represent a secure base and the interpersonal space necessary for the therapeutic process. My therapeutic experience shows that this process is only possible if my mental state is one of collaboration and I manage to express my *compassion* toward my client. I felt no difficulty in expressing my compassion toward Maria, although she did have a deficit of compassion toward herself that she took from her family of origin and from all the psychological baggage she carried.

Maria, now 50 years old, had some challenges in deciphering nonverbal messages and signals that came from her interlocutor; in other words, she had trouble with *contingent* communication, a way in which the signals of one person are perceived, made sense of, and responded to in a timely and effective manner (Siegel, 2012). This made her feel stuck in her sense of communication and attunement both in her private relationship and her professional ones. We approached this issue through a series of pendulations between her present difficulties and the recollection of childhood experiences which facilitated the process of self-discovery and self-awareness.

Following some behavioral prescriptions, Maria was encouraged to have conversations with her mother (her only living parent) about the experiences in the past and the transgenerational baggage of her family. Through these conversations, she found out that during the Second World War her grandmother had been the victim of rape and her mother (who had been just a little child) assisted in this act of cruelty done by one of the soldiers. It is not by chance, thus, that Maria's mother ended up working in the police force and then in the SRI (Romanian Services of Information). Awareness of this history helped Maria get a bit of clearance and understanding regarding her fundamental anxiety and look toward the "inner child" within her mother, which illustrates the systemic connections across her, her mother, her grandmother, and sociocultural trauma contexts.

Acquiring a sense of knowledge and meaning ended up having a positive influence on Maria's self-esteem and the improvement of our relationship determined a certain *cohesion*. During the entire process of therapy, which lasted about a year and a half, the contingent connection and the discovery of some of the secrets in her family system (the family of origin) favored a deeper feeling of *continuity*, which ended up representing a repairing system for intergenerational ruptures.

All these combined (the connection of the therapeutic space, the compassion in this space, improved contingency, psychological cohesion in the here and now, and the *coherence* of what happens) helped Maria to gain a certain *clarity* of herself and her system of reference. Going back to her family of origin and the conversations with her mother led to more shared experiences and to what Siegel (2003) called *co-construction* or co-creation of a life story. The complexity of such intervention, which targets both the work we do in the practice space and redefines the connection with the family of origin, sums up the *complexity* that stands for healing and freeing oneself from the burden of the past.

The changes were visible as Maria showed a deeper and more mature *self-awareness*, which was to become her secure base in the here and now, protecting her from the psychological regressions in the past. And the energy she saved by leaving the past in the past and by making its intrusions less present was used by Maria to expand her *creativity* and cultivate her vitality. At the beginning of therapy, Maria was withdrawn and socially isolated; after the therapeutic process, she became more and more open toward the people around her, cultivating some solid friendships and a more authentic anchoring in the *community* she is part of. Once she managed to build this courage to connect, Maria felt not only her relationship with herself take shape, but also the feeling of belonging to her family and her community started to flourish. Just as Siegel (2003) said, finding a sense of belonging is a process that develops more and more as we manage to overcome the boundaries of our skin.

In the process of therapeutic intervention with Maria, the keys were the connection and her courage to discover the unknown history of her family through the eyes of the adult she became, and her deeper awareness of how the present and the past mixed up helped her gain a sense of mastery over her person and, thus, live more in the "here and now." This shows us, again and again, that both the connection and the discovery of the truth free us from the chains of trauma and offer us the chance to bloom and thrive.

Clinical Implications

A needed prerequisite for the healing of trauma for the people of Romania lies in access to good psychotherapy services. But, my professional experience and conversations with colleagues all over the country show me that not everything can be solved by offering services as usual; a great impact is given by the paradigm of the therapists. Are they willing/able to take into account the history of the client? Can they see these problems through a sociocultural lens? Does the therapist have a systemic or relational approach? After more than a decade and a half of working in this area, I can say that focusing on the content but ignoring the context is likely to be useless and can even become harmful. The therapist must not only have an arsenal of valuable techniques for intervention, but also a socioculturally attuned perspective that constantly explores the connections between the micro-systems (client, couple, family) and macro-systems (community, city, region, country).

A relational view sees the "mind" as not only something physiological within an individual brain, but also as happening *between* people (Siegel, 2019). And, the embodied brain, interpersonal relationships, and the larger social world reciprocally create each other. According to Siegel, "a healthy mind is a mind that creates integration within the body and its brain, and within relationships with other people and the planet" (p. 227). When the flow of energy and information between these components is blocked, as is the case in the Romanian collective experience, personal, relational, and societal health is not possible. Instead, people's responses to one another and to life's circumstances are either chaotic or rigid. Our job as therapists is to promote the integration of the inner and inter aspects of the mind.

When we attune to the internal state of another with compassion, neural integration is stimulated for each person. In other words, "relational integration stimulates the growth of integration in the brain" (Siegel, 2019, p. 230). To establish a good therapeutic relationship, the client needs to recognize and understand the necessity of engaging in the healing process, and the therapist needs to express compassion toward the subjective experiences of the client.

Thus, the trust that gets created between the two, client and psychotherapist, leads to the further creation of psychological cohesion, and coming to successive sessions ensures continuity. All of this will lead to a deeper sense of coherence about what is happening in the inner universe of the client. The co-creation of shared experiences that can happen both through verbal and nonverbal communication is dependent on clarity and communion. And the complexity that results from this kind of resonance between two or more people determines a neuronal integration or, better said, deeper healing. Resonance implies a mutual influence between the two people and ensures the presence of one in the mind of the other, even when the two people are not together.

Having made such a psychological journey, both an inner journey and an interpersonal one, Romanians could have greater access to their mental resources such as creativity and intelligence, getting to enjoy their true complexity. The entire process could enhance courage toward interpersonal connection and could reconstruct a sense of community. I think that, in many ways, finding the value of interpersonal connection is the equivalent of finding the meaning of human existence.

For those of us who will not find the necessary willpower to undertake such a transformational journey, some trauma experts such as Drs. Peter Levine (2010, 2022), Gábor Maté (2004, 2021), and Bassel van der Kolk (2015) remind us that psychotherapy is not the only way. Since trauma is experienced in the body, the body is a place where one can find sources of its healing. To do this, we need to identify the proper context that could support us in hearing the unspoken voice of the human body. Activities such as yoga, techniques of recognition and acceptance of bodily sensations, breathing exercises, body therapies, or some traditional spiritual practices can be of great benefit in this sense. All of these can help us in reconnecting with our Self and can represent an important step in our healing process. And if we accept the relational side of ourselves, the next step will take us closer to the world we're a part of.

Conclusion

We are born in relationships, we live in relationships, we get hurt in relationships, and we heal in relationships (Hendrix & LaKelly Hunt, 2021). Some of us use the power of relationships as a portal getting us closer to our souls, and others start their journey toward this interpersonal space driven by spiritual or shamanic wisdom. In my book, *Souls of Glass* (Gáspár, 2020), a combination of fiction and psychology based on scientific evidence, I present the complicated story of a couple who are child adults. Two young people who carry in their respective emotional baggage various traumas and who fear intimacy deeply. To better help the reader understand the psychology of trauma, I present the story of two by offering various examples from real-life borrowed from the experience of the clients I worked with, from my personal life, and that of my family of origin. Again, to stay open to the various healing possibilities, only one of the characters is helped by undergoing a process of individual psychotherapy, while the other uses yoga practice, after which gets attracted by the infinite opportunities offered by psychodrama.

To promote relational health in Romania, in 2012 my colleagues and I set up a training school for family psychotherapy with the mission to promote what we named #RelationalRevolutionInRomania (#RevoluțiaRelaționalăÎnRomânia). We offer complimentary training courses in relational psychotherapy, publish renowned international authors, and have an educational platform through which we organize conferences and scientific events. The journey is long—after all, only a decade has passed since we started to consciously promote relational health in Romania, but more and more of us now know that the quality of our life depends on the quality of our relationships.

What humanity can learn from the story of the Romanian people is that trauma affects relationships; it sabotages both the connection we have with ourselves and the trust we have in others. As Thomas Hübl (2020) stated in *Healing Collective Trauma*, at a collective level traumatic dysregulation is mainly cultural and generational. When we want to see, we can easily notice how our close ones—partners, children, parents, friends, colleagues, and neighbors—manage their psychological–biological energy. Is there a connection with self and anchoring in their own life or are they in a perpetual energy mobile? When we start to befriend our energy and gain some somatic awareness, the process will be visible to those around us, but just as visible is the disconnection from our own body, emotions, and relational system of which we're part. The degree of disconnection mirrors our inner suffering and our interpersonal suffering, and in crises, the magnitude of suffering gets enhanced at a personal and a sociocultural level.

Romanians, and probably the whole of humanity, are at the point in which its future relies on this collective healing. Our well-being lies in interpersonal security, and the legacy we leave to future generations relies on what we do now. When we will be able to find (again) the road toward mutual support and we realize that the connections (relationships) between us are more important than we may believe, and when we will dare to offer the painful memories due importance, we will realize, for real, the power that our relationships hold—in the family, in the community, and the entire world. Only then will our ancestors be able to rest, and our descendants will be able to prosper. For this entire script to represent more than just a psychological process described in a book, the Romanian people need to dare make the first steps toward an unknown territory—one in which they could safely explore their past, traumas, and emotions, and be rewarded with the gift of psychological flexibility (i.e., moving from cognitive rigidity and mental chaos).

Is healing possible? Without a doubt: yes! The science of relationality and interpersonal neurobiology provides an answer. Our self is profoundly relational. Even more, we cannot function outside a relational system. Are the Romanian people capable of reinventing themselves and regaining their interpersonal peace? I dare say yes. All that is left to do is to remind ourselves who we are, what we are dealing with, and what we want to pass on.

References

David, D. (2015). *Psihologia poporului român*. Editura Polirom.

Eger, E. (2021). *Darul*. Editura Trei.

Gáspár, G. (2020). *Suflete de sticlă*. Pagina de Psihologie.

Hendrix, H., & LaKelly Hunt, H. (2021). *Doing imago relationship therapy*. W.W. Norton & Company.

Hübl, T. (2020). *Healing collective trauma*. Sounds True.

Institutul Naţional de Statistică. (2022). *Demographic events in 2021*. https://insse.ro/cms/en/content/demographic-events-202

Levine, P. A. (2010). *In an unspoken voice: How the body releases trauma and restores goodness*. North Atlantic Books.

Levine, P. (2022). *Într-o voce nerostită*. Pagina de Psihologie.

Maté, G. (2004). *When the body says no: The hidden cost of stress*. Knoph.

Maté, G. (2021). *Când corpul spune nu*. Curtea Veche.

Miller, A. (2019). *Drama copilului interior*. Herald.

Siegel, D. J. (2003). An interpersonal neurobiology of psychotherapy: The developing mind and the resolution of trauma. In M. F. Solomon & D. J. Siegel (Eds.), *Healing trauma: Attachment, mind, body, and brain* (pp. 1–56). W.W. Norton & Company.

Siegel, D. J. (2012). *Pocket guide to interpersonal neurobiology*. W.W. Norton & Company.

Siegel, D. J. (2018). *Mintea*. Pagina de Psihologie.

Siegel, D. J. (2019). The mind in psychotherapy: An interpersonal neurobiology framework for understanding and cultivating mental health. *Psychology and Psychotherapy: Theory, Research and Practice, 92*, 224–237.

Solomon, M. F., & Siegel, D. J. (2003). *Healing trauma: Attachment, mind, body, and brain*. W.W. Norton & Company.

van der Kolk, B. (2015). *The body keeps the score*. Penguin Random House.

Chapter 5
Sociocultural Trauma Among Marginalized Families in Moldova

Valentina Bodrug-Lungu, Natalia Toma, and Sergiu Toma

We are specialists in family issues and family therapy with teaching and clinical practice experience who live and work in Moldova, a country bordered by Ukraine and Romania. As we write, we are acutely aware that the people of Moldova have a history of significant sociocultural trauma that is once again reactivated by the invasion of Ukraine.

Brief Country Overview

Moldova, officially the Republic of Moldova, is a country in Eastern Europe. Moldova emerged as an independent republic following the collapse of the Soviet Union in 1991 (see Maps 3 and 4, Appendix, this volume). Moldova is considered one of the poorest countries in Europe, with its economy relying heavily on agriculture (BBC, 2021). At the same time, despite several challenges, according to official sources (Government of the Republic of Moldova, 2020), the Republic of Moldova is continuously advancing a domestic reform agenda and aligning to European standards.

The Republic of Moldova ranked 90 out of 189 countries and territories in the UNDP's (2020) latest Global Human Development Index, HDI 2019, which put the country in the high human development category. Between 1990 and 2019, life expectancy at birth increased by 4.3 years and mean years of schooling increased by 3.7 years. Gross National Income per capita decreased by about 3.6% (UNDP, 2020).

V. Bodrug-Lungu (✉) · N. Toma · S. Toma
Moldova State University, Chisinau, Moldova
e-mail: valentina.bodrug.lungu@usm.md

T. Glebova, C. Knudson-Martin (eds.), *Sociocultural Trauma and Well-Being in Eastern European Family Therapy*, AFTA SpringerBriefs in Family Therapy,
https://doi.org/10.1007/978-3-031-29995-7_5

The Republic of Moldova has signed and ratified all relevant international legal frameworks pertaining to human rights, including gender equality and the empowerment of women. The country's legislative and normative frameworks in support of gender equality and advancing women's empowerment are relatively strong. Despite this progress, implementation of this legal framework remains a significant challenge.

Demographic Profile

According to the latest studies, the Republic of Moldova is undergoing profound demographic changes related to declining population numbers, continuous aging, low fertility, emigration of the able-bodied population, and low life expectancy (UNFPA, 2022). Since the proclamation of independence in 1991, Moldova has lost about 1.5 million people out of about four million at the time of detachment from the USSR. Most have left in recent years. Moldova loses 45,000 citizens annually, most of them economically active young people who are looking for stability and opportunities to build their future. Most have left the Transnistrian region, where, in addition to poverty, the population also faces an authoritarian, pro-Russian separatist regime based on corruption (DW, 2022).

As of January 1, 2021, the Republic of Moldova was one of the smallest countries in Europe with a population of 2.597 million, which consists of 52.2% women and 47.8% men. The coefficient of population aging is 22.5 people aged 60 and over per 100 inhabitants in 2021, with a strong prevalence of women (NBS, 2021).

Socioeconomic Conditions

The absolute poverty rate gradually declined from 29.5% in 2014 to 26.8% in 2020, with the poverty rate higher where the head of the household is a woman (NBS, 2020). The proportion of the population below the international poverty line of US$4.3 per day decreased, with significant differences between rural and urban populations. Despite some progress, the labor market faces multiple challenges, including low wages, poor quality of employment, informal employment, and labor migration processes. Women with children have fewer economic opportunities compared to men.

Education

While Moldova has made important progress in nearly universal enrollment of both boys and girls in primary and secondary education, the proportion of female graduates of higher education has remained around 60% since 2009. Moreover, the number of young people in Moldovan universities has halved since then. Every year 4500 young people between the ages of 19 and 24 leave to go abroad (DW, 2022).

Women's Empowerment

Moldova's legal and regulatory frameworks in support of gender equality and women's empowerment are relatively strong: the 1994 National Constitution prohibits discrimination (art.32 (3)) and stipulates the equality of citizens before the law regardless of nationality, religion, sex, etc. (Constitution, 2022, art.16 (2)). In 2006, the Law on Equal Opportunities for Women and Men was adopted. Women's representation in the national Parliament gradually increased from 8.9% in 1998–2000 to 39.6% in July 2021. Women's leadership roles also increased at the local level; the proportion of elected women mayors was 10.9% in 1999 and 21.8% in 2019 (UN Women, 2021). Despite the progress, women continue to face multiple socioeconomic problems.

A number of statistical indicators reveal sociodemographic differences between rural and urban women. Rural women in Moldova face reduced access to facilities, poor quality of services, and lack of employment opportunities, among others. Due to low fertility and labor migration, there is a significant share of single elderly women in villages, who "survive" given the reduced opportunities to generate income for subsistence (low pensions, heavy land works). The sociodemographic trends described above are rooted in past sociocultural traumatic experiences by the people of Moldova.

Moldova's Experience of Sociocultural Trauma

The proclamation of the country's independence in 1991 led to the exit from the Soviet Union. This was a crucial and prescribed societal change from a totalitarian regime to a democratic society in all areas of the society: political, economic, social, and cultural, which caused drastic transformation. Communist totalitarian societies and the trauma of its sudden collapse have led to mixed emotional reactions, from being glad and satisfied with the opportunity to rebuild the sense of national cultural identity to feeling anxious, conflict avoidant, and somewhat lost.

The Republic of Moldova's experience of sociocultural trauma is various. Among the most powerful events that had a traumatic impact on individuals and society as a whole are the military conflict in Transnistria, the war in Ukraine, economic migration, and the trauma of communism and the social change that followed in the post-communist societies.

Military Conflict in the Transnistria Region

The proclamation of the country's independence also led to the outbreak of military conflict in the Transnistria region in 1992, which is currently in latency. During the years after the armed conflict, the negotiation process used as the main tool for resolving the Transnistrian problem did not lead to its settlement.

One aspect of war trauma refers to soldiers that were directly involved in the military actions as well as their family members: mothers that lost their sons, women that lost their husbands, and children that lost their dads or witnessed their distress after returning from war. Though a good part of the active participants in the military actions (police, military) have benefited from some rehabilitation assistance, their families had to deal with everything by themselves.

Another significant element of this military conflict was ethnic tension being provoked in the context of disputes regarding national identity, primarily between Russian and Moldovan citizens. Thus, the patriotic feelings and cultural liberation somewhat regained after the independence from the communist regime was replaced by a sense of uncertainty, anxiety, and mistrust in the Moldovan government's ability to protect its citizens from another trauma (war) and vulnerability due to its inability to care for them during and after the traumatic event. The current context of the war in Ukraine has triggered a similar reaction among Moldovan citizens and those that live in the Transnistrian region that in a possible military action of Russia in Moldova, part of the citizens from the Transnistrian region may associate with Russia while on the right bank of the Dniester many men of different ages prefer to leave the country rather than fight for sovereignty (findings based on the analysis of social media).

Currently, beyond the political debates about sovereignty between the government of the Republic of Moldova and the separatist regime in Transnistria, the split in opinions is maintained at the level of individuals, families, and society: some being oriented toward Europe, others toward Russia. Here we find an intersection between the current war trauma and other sociopolitical traumas related to national identity, the Soviet past through the provision of social protection, etc. The following case illustrates this.

Testimony from a Veteran from the 1992 Transnistria Conflict

What started on February 24, 2022, but rather in the evening at 18:30 on February 23, when the first rockets were launched on Ukraine ... Has terrified me and a lot of people were forced to leave their houses, having to flee from the fury. I personally saw this on the very day of March 1, 1992, voluntarily walking across the bridge from Vadul lui Vodă and seeing those extraordinarily large columns, frightened eyes, frightened children. What I saw in 92 I still remember today. Unfortunately, it is an unlearned lesson of the events in Transnistria from 1991–1999.

The War in Ukraine

The dramatic events happening in Ukraine forced millions of people to flee and leave their homes. Thousands of Ukrainians came across the Ukrainian–Moldovan border, and remained here, keeping a hope to come back home one day. These events required mental health professionals to help the refugees face the traumatic events they are living through. Every refugee is affected in some way by the situations of injury or witness of injuries or death of other people. Many of the refugees that came to Moldova have experienced typical PTSD symptoms and tended to see Moldova as a transit destination due to its economic, military, and geographical vulnerability. Also, the war and the narrative of it promoted by the Russian government have reactivated collective sociocultural trauma from the collapse of the Soviet Union (followed by the conflict in Transnistria) and reclaiming independence. Moldovan citizens almost instantly felt fear, denial, uncertainty, and anger expressed in the need to find a safer place. The war in Ukraine has forced some Moldovans to consider leaving the country.

Testimony from a Ukrainian refugee displaced in Moldova
From the first days of the war I couldn't sleep or eat for 3 days, It's like the stories of my grandfathers from the second world war. I came to Moldova because I have many friends here and in Poland; my grandmother is Polish. In fact, we are one brotherly people with Moldovans. Now, our people are showing great unity, especially now, when it is an extremely difficult situation. I believe that we have never been so united.

Migration Processes

Moldova is significantly affected by migration processes. The flow of the emigrant population increased from about 700 thousand in 2014 to 1159 thousand in 2020 (UNFPA, 2022). It has a controversial impact. On the one hand, the remittances sent home by migrants have contributed to not only the improvement of the socioeconomic situation of the relatives but also of the society as a whole. On the other hand, migration, among other factors, contributes to depopulation, especially in rural areas, intensification of aging processes, high rates of divorce and gender imbalances, particularly in the reproductive age group, threatens the sustainability of pension systems, and has a negative impact on the labor market. Due to the fact that migration differentially affected various population groups (in Moldova and abroad) and connected closely with family issues related to children and the older population, this represents another type of trauma manifested by suffering, anxiety, alcohol/ psychotropic substances abuse, low self-esteem, etc. As a result of trauma prior and during migration, women frequently experienced psychosomatic symptoms such as headaches, anxiety, insomnia, and loss of appetite.

Migration has been significantly forced and can be correlated with the overall societal discord and lack of national unity created by political leaders, which have exploited the communist ideas among Russian speaking citizens and those matured in the former Soviet Union and that have been disappointed by democratic governments that have failed to keep their promises. All this sociopolitical trauma of having leaders that are governed from outside the country and therefore are an expression of the communist government model have triggered reactions of flight or fight. This has forced a sense of disappointment and lack of a reliably democratic vision for many citizens, especially among the young generations. After more than a decade of pro-communist leadership that have not kept their promises and made no significant changes, in July 2021, due to the massive mobilization of the diaspora against the socialist regime (pro-Russian, connected to the Soviet historical past), the political regime was changed, with pro-European forces coming to Governance.

Clinical Responses to Sociocultural Trauma

As illustrated in Chap. 1 (Glebova et al., this volume), sociocultural trauma has both immediate and long-term impacts. Each is relevant today in Moldova as clinicians and other support workers respond to the psychological and interpersonal effects resulting from the war in Ukraine and longer-term trauma related to sudden political change, uncertainty, and division, including domestic violence and the impact of COVID-19.

Immediate Crisis Intervention

Primary psychological care and intervention in crisis situations, such as the impact of the war in Ukraine, refer to the measures taken to identify those affected by trauma and help them overcome the shock caused by the traumatic event and adapt to environmental demands, as well as facilitating connection with other specialized services such as medical care, psychiatric consultation, and community support. Such emergency psychological supports are directed toward restoring a person's level of competence and adaptive functioning and preventing or reducing the negative impact of the traumatic event to which they were subjected and providing information about adaptive coping methods and possible reactions to stress through psychoeducation.

Children are especially vulnerable in crisis situations. Traumatic events destroy safety in the universe in which they live—their favorite places and things—and disrupt their routine activities, shatter their dreams, and impair confidence in adults. In the chaos caused by the crisis situation, children may be further traumatized by malicious adults/criminals and more exposed to the risk of violence and psychological, physical, or sexual abuse. Also, adults overwhelmed by looking for solutions for physical survival (shelter, food, water, and hygiene) may ignore the emotional needs of children, which aggravates their situation.

Several organizations (Institute for Family and Social Initiative from Moldova, Gender-Centru, and others) mobilized volunteers to provide emotional support to children and to provide play and reading activities to minimize the effects of traumatic events. Primary psychological assistance such as this should be directed toward evaluation of basic needs and worries, listening without forcing them to speak, and consolation. The following principles are foundational to crisis intervention:

- All actions must be aimed at avoiding any potential danger and physical or psychological harm to the people helped.
- Treat assisted people with utmost respect and discretion, trying to conform to their cultural and social norms, gender, age, etc. and ensuring that people can access help without discrimination.
- Assist people in claiming and obtaining rights and access to available aid. Act only in the best interest of the assisted person.

When addressing a person in crisis, it is important to stay calm and have a gentle and calm tone. If it is culturally appropriate, maintain eye contact. If someone feels that what is happening to them is unrealistic or seems disconnected from their environment, it may be helpful for them to have contact with their current environment and themselves, for example, by washing their face with water. We can invite the person to touch us, to shake our hands as tightly as possible. People in crisis can also be helped by asking them to do the following, "Put your feet down and feel the contact with the ground. Trot with your feet. Press your fingers or hands on your knees. Observe elements in the environment, such as things you see, hear, or feel—please tell us what you see."

Intersection of Sociocultural Trauma and Domestic Violence

Domestic violence (DV), which encompasses a wide range of behaviors that use physical, psychological, and/or economic force to injure or abuse family members, is one-way sociocultural trauma manifests itself. DV-related trauma is disproportionately experienced by certain groups because of deeply entrenched structural inequalities, with gender inequality a key determinant of violence against women. Additional risk factors for DV are alcohol and drug use, which are often culturally approved self-medication of trauma, and past experiences of violent victimization. PTSD is also associated with an increased risk of violence. A poor socioeconomic environment can exacerbate stress and inability to cope with problems, which in turn result in acts of violence.

Domestic violence survivors often face ongoing and challenging effects of abuse. People who have experienced trauma as a result of a family member often report shame, guilt, and high levels of depression and anxiety, which add to sociocultural-based uncertainty and silence around shared sociocultural trauma. According to official data, violence against women is one of the most prevalent forms of violence in Moldova. Two in five women (40%) say they have experienced physical and/or sexual violence at the hands of a partner or nonpartner since the age of 15 (OSCE, 2019).

During the pandemic, the prevalence of physical violence increased, especially toward women and children. Escaping an abusive environment generated by someone who is expected to care, protect, and share responsibilities is challenging in a social context where abuse is part of a cultural history toward women and is an ongoing struggle, especially during a health crisis. In our experience, high rates of DV are both a consequence of complex sociocultural trauma and perpetuate it.

DV is related to insidious gender inequality at the societal level. Research suggests that the success of ending violence is a hard-to-obtain goal, especially if considered only at the individual level; there is a need for comprehensive interdisciplinary measures at all levels of society, with a strong focus on prevention programs. Services should be carefully designed with sensitivity to gender inequality and must counteract cultural historical imprints at the individual level and a sense of guilt for women for speaking or fighting against violence. The paradigms guiding DV services need to also be sensitive to and address intergenerational trauma and rigid views of gender roles. The goals that are broadly applicable to most therapeutic approaches are to support the survivors to regain safety or some personal security strategies, together with decreasing negative symptoms such as fear, anxiety, sleep disorder, etc. and as a long-term goal, support survivors to regain relational and personal trust, while becoming more aware of risks for abuse and establishing clearer relational boundaries that will allow a person to feel safe and confident as relationships unfold, especially with intimate partners.

Support for Trauma Victims

In the Republic of Moldova, identification of post-traumatic stress disorder (PTSD) by doctors or clinical psychologists is rare, and the rehabilitation process is long, difficult, and costly for victims, their families, and society as a whole (Popovici, 2019). Most services are currently supported by nonprofit organizations specialized in domestic violence. The broad set of symptoms that need to be addressed include feelings of guilt about the specific role of the victim; distrust of one's own strength and that of others caused by abuse (physical, psychological or financial); difficulties in relating to the family of origin; fear and anger as a result of violence; relationship with the aggressor (wealth sharing, children's visit schedule, etc.); lack of functional coping mechanisms in situations of emotional crisis; shame related to motherhood; and lack of emotional resources to achieve personal goals. Often, the symptoms (especially the distrust of one's own strength and difficulties in relating to the family of origin) are related and amplified by the sociocultural trauma; victims report persistence over their lifetimes as a typical and even transgenerational experience of abuse, particularly in an uncertain societal context.

Effective psychological support when dealing with traumatic events at the individual level moves from providing safety to reconnecting with supportive others and understanding and redefining norms based on socioculturally reinforced trauma. These goals include the following:

- Establishing a safe environment for the person affected by trauma.
- Considering the emotional and behavioral reactions described above as a result of trauma and framing them as survival coping strategies.
- Reconnecting for support and understanding with persons that were distanced by the traumatic experiences or finding new relationships that can fulfill this need.
- Integrating the traumatic experience into a personal and/or family history that allows growth and further development.

"I feel more confident after psychotherapy and especially the support group I have been part of."

"I have learned to be more in control of myself, to appreciate myself, to leave the past in the past, and not to be ashamed by what people will say about me, my family, and my decision to leave the abusive relationship or any other relationships where I am not treated properly."

"I am more aware of the fact that it was not only about me, it was about my past experiences and what I have been taught to view and accept as normal. But now I have a different view—Abuse is not normal."

Source: Survivor of sexual abuse from an intimate partner. Feedback from a final stage of psychotherapy at the NGO Institute for Family and Social Initiative from Moldova (from a program that provided psychotherapy for women affected by abuse and domestic violence)

COVID–19 Impact

The COVID-19 pandemic also had a major impact on the population's perception of safety. Not only were usual interpersonal behaviors constrained, human rights in Moldova were also limited, especially for the most vulnerable groups (youth, persons with disabilities, and elderly people).

Data (Covrig et al., 2020) indicate that 20% of young people in Moldova reported a worsening of their psychological well-being during the pandemic crisis, compared to before (January–February of 2020). The negative effects of isolation measures have been most pronounced on girls, young people in urban areas, and those on low incomes (Covrig et al., 2020). According to this research, the impact of the pandemic was revealed through emotional negative symptoms (sadness, fear, crying) and physical well-being (insomnia, loss of appetite, headache).

Though official data do not reveal the connection between the prevalence of reported symptoms and the overall social context, there is a higher tendency in reported symptoms among young people that have requested professional support from families with vulnerability (one or both parents working abroad, living with grandparents, history of abuse and separation/divorce), which suggests that the degree of sociocultural safety is an important factor affecting how people responded to the COVID-19 issues.

Dissatisfaction with one's own way of life, social isolation, and distance measures, in turn, exacerbated risky behaviors. The pandemic crisis triggered a series of changes both in terms of attitudes/self-perceptions and behavior. Isolation restrictions and distancing from the social environment have led to a worsening of the situation regarding the consumption of alcohol and tobacco and other practices harmful to health (beatings, drunk driving, self-harm), especially among boys. Thus, out of the total number of young people who smoked cigarettes in the last 12 months, about 37% used tobacco much more often during the crisis (Covrig et al., 2020), which indirectly indicates the state of emotional tension and stress among them.

Despite the high level of anxiety during the pandemic, few young people enlisted the help of professionals. Most young people preferred to seek support from their own community contexts (family, relatives, friends) and less from people who could have provided specialized/professional services. Although there are no significant differences in behavior between girls and boys, we do notice a slightly higher tendency among girls to use specialized services. At the same time, we attested a higher level of vulnerability in rural areas, where there was no evidence of endorsement for professional support, compared to 8% in the case of young people in urban areas.

While the ongoing COVID-19 pandemic has had traumatic consequences in Moldova and added additional anxiety, depression, and suffering to the social uncertainties and disease already prevalent at the societal level, in our context, the pandemic and its aftermath also offer opportunity—lessons learned on how to survive together and adjust to new conditions, to remake the world as well as to live in it.

Opportunities for Sociocultural Change

A large proportion of families in Moldova are facing the consequences of intergenerational trauma with cultural and historical premises, which often can be signaled by high tolerance to abuse, a family history of loss, separation as a consequence of abuse, death, or suicide. Current social perceptions regarding gender roles and tolerance of abuse create a social context of high social and economic vulnerability for women. Men also experience multiple risk factors, such as low opportunities to be perceived as heroic, successful, or self-confident when performing parental roles, or even to be seen as competent enough in the context of a new legal framework that supports a more egalitarian view of the society.

During recent years, especially due to the increased mobility of the population, there are changes in the cultural context of the Republic of Moldova, which is characterized by a symbiosis of traditional patriarchal norms with modern values. The current situation can be characterized as a balance between traditionalism and modernism. These changes are a challenge, given that historically the traditional family was considered the supreme value. The sociocultural and political changes in relation to the family have affected all generations, but mostly the elderly, especially from rural areas. We find the intersection of sociocultural, political, and intergenerational trauma through suffering and diminishing family relationships, but with different gender and intergenerational impacts. More than that, the emphasis in the more recent third wave of migration is that family members from Moldova move to their relatives or family members already living abroad as a family reunification.

At the same time, many times, the values related to physical and economic survival have a higher priority than democracy, free choice, and autonomy, especially for the adult population and the elderly. All this has its roots in the experience from the historical past related to the Soviet system, when the mentioned "values" were falsely opposed to democracy. We must recognize that the current traumatic social factors (suffering and dissatisfaction with the social protection system and medical care, low pensions), formed during the years of independence, intersect with sociopolitical trauma, linked to political instability, corruption, and economic inefficiency of governments. The challenge remains the nostalgia of many elderly people for a "strong" government of the past (Stalinist, which maintained public order), social protection, and medical assistance provided by the state.

Recommendations for Clinical Practice

Moving beyond an individual frame to include a sociocultural one enables people to address the interpersonal and social challenges and contradictions inherent in a changing sociopolitical environment. We highlight engaging fathers and the value of group work as two clinical practices that create the opportunity to help transform societal norms and expectations and build relational resilience that enables people to better deal with uncertainties, tension, and conflict in the larger society.

Engaging Parents—Especially Fathers

Though people in Moldova value two-parent families and fathers remain involved with their children to some extent, clinicians readily excuse fathers from attending appointments due to work commitments or because they are not the primary caretakers of their children. However, the social contextual factors described above point to the need for family therapists and clinicians to emphasize the engagement of fathers or both parents regardless of marital status and to also look at internalized models of intimate family relationships when thinking about change in dyadic interaction patterns. In turn, this relates to children's socioemotional adaptation and overcoming traumatic experiences such that new, more equitable relational possibilities and expectations can evolve.

Engaging both parents (especially men/fathers) can be of specific utility in exploring the consequences of sociocultural trauma due to the range of symptoms reported by fathers—guilt for being obligated to be the only breadwinner, fear of being perceived as incompetent when dealing with children, anger and frustration of being unable to take care of children, and sense of isolation, loneliness, and fear of rejection when manifesting vulnerability. We recommend inviting both mothers and fathers to reflect on their specific family and social traumatic context and build a strength-based approach when planning interventions. Some practical questions may be: *What is your family history of father engagement? What stories were told behind the father's absence from home/education? How often have other men expressed their fears and vulnerabilities? What traumatic contexts (family and societal) led to the rigid separation of family roles by men and women* (e.g., *death, war, abuse, illness,* etc.)*? What parental behaviors were and still are verbally encouraged for men?* These questions can lead to a broad range of insights that can link the reported symptoms to a broader understanding through the lens of sociocultural trauma, both in men as fathers and among other family members. Organizing individual sessions with men can facilitate further collaboration in working through traumatic issues.

This shift in clinical practice can be especially beneficial because adoption of a preventive approach to male emotional and physical health will emphasize the therapeutic advantages of earlier problem recognition and appropriate help-seeking action for men and boys and also strengthen their parenting competences (Heubeck et al., 1986). As for women, the shift can be a unique opportunity to renegotiate responsibilities and be more aware of the specific benefits of father engagement, not only in trauma therapy, but for child development and relational life in general.

Some beliefs often held about children by their parents are particularly ripe for questioning, especially those that contribute to the blunting of boys' sensitivity and later resentment expressed through the abuse of physical power. Examples of implicit beliefs we raise for explicit questioning include: Is it alright for children to be 'indulged'? Will praise make children big-headed? Will gentleness make boys less able to deal with the world? Will 'softness' make boys less popular with women as adults, or incline them toward being gay? Why are we so afraid of gay men? If it is alright for boys to be upset, is it equally alright for them to show their feelings—and to their fathers as well? Are their fathers likely to be available for them (physically and emotionally)? Can you like a crying boy (over the age of four)? Can we give children a balanced view of the importance of the world of relationships with people and the world of relationships with things? (Walters et al., 2001).

Group Therapy and Support Groups

Research emphasizes the effectiveness of group therapy due to its ability to simulate small-scale societal healing through shared experience and transformation as persons simultaneously individually and collectively come to a point of recognizing the importance of each other in their personal change. We consider this approach to be partially validated by practice in the Republic of Moldova that shows similar conclusions as prior research (Cacciatore, 2007). Quantitative results utilizing the *Impact of Event Scale Revised* demonstrate that women who attend support groups, when controlling for time, had fewer post-traumatic stress symptoms than did the women who did not attend a support group. Qualitative results elucidate the role of support groups in managing grief, suggesting that connectivity with other women may be a useful strategy in reducing problematic psychological outcomes (Cacciatore, 2007).

The particular benefits of group therapy for sociocultural trauma are the opportunities to reflect on the social context and use the group dynamics to integrate the individual symptoms in broader social context that leads to less isolation, social disengagement (specific to PTSD), and a much deeper understanding of the influence of the social context. Group therapy also enables people to connect with sources of resilience within themselves and others. By providing an alternative relational experience in which the survivor and their safety are valued, groups empower members to establish self-affirming and supportive relationships in their outside lives.

When delivering group therapy, there is obviously a need to specify the format of the group (open or closed, time limited with a specific set of themes depending on different circumstances), though some positive practices conclude that the closed and time-limited ones have a better consideration in the cultural context. Feedback from participants in support groups for survivors of domestic violence provided by the Institute for Family and Social Initiatives suggests the following as helpful topics to explore (IFIS, 2021):

- Setting personal goals—Me and the others.
- The circle of trust and security—Increasing self-confidence and boundaries.
- Reconsidering the traumatic events (violence, divorce, separation)—View of the society and family history of trauma.
- The work of loss and acceptance—Exploring the stage each is at.
- Forgiveness—Self and other.

- Reconnecting with oneself and others.
- Envisioning change and planning for the future.

Group Therapy Case Example

Maria, aged 43, came to the group sessions after a period on individual sessions with a psychologist following a family crisis that led to several years of experiencing intimate partner violence and community shaming: *"My mother and grandmother used to say: If something bad is happening in the family, it's only the women's responsibility; they are the ones that provide harmony and if there is no harmony there is a bad wife. You need to have fear from your man—Without him you are nothing. Group therapy made me realize that most women share my sense of guilt, self-blame, and a deep sense of feeling alone when you are hurt in the family; maybe this is a story for many women in Moldova who decided to keep quiet, who are faced with poverty, uncertainty of the future, and fatherlessness."* during the group sessions Maria came to realize that the community history of most of the women she knew was of physical abuse, which was something everyone knew but nobody was willing to name. Together they began to develop a new story of what it means to be a woman.

Conclusions

Moldova has an ongoing history of political, economic, and demographic vulnerability and a history of sociocultural trauma as a result of the impacts of communism, post-communist transition, and war. Women and men have been struggling with rigid societal expectations that have triggered and maintained violence toward children, women, and men. Overcoming these dangerous effects of a large-scale phenomenon at the individual level requires seeing family relationships as a place of change, safety, and choice. Exploring possibilities through family and group therapy and prompt crisis interventions can provide comprehensive guidance to transforming social and cultural influences on individual and relational well-being.

References

BBC. (2021). Moldova country profile https://www.bbc.com/news/world-europe-17601580

Cacciatore, J. (2007). Effects of support groups on post-traumatic stress responses in women. Experiencing Stillbirth https://journals.sagepub.com/doi/abs/10.2190/M447-1X11-6566-8042

Constitution of the Republic of Moldova. (2022). https://www.parlament.md/CadrulLegal/Constitution/tabid/151/language/en-US/Default.aspx

Covrig, N., Buzu, A. & Cantarji, V. (2020). COVID-19 și tinerii: Efectele pandemiei asupra bunăstării psiho-emoționale [COVID-19 and young people: The effects of the pandemic on welfare psycho-emotional]. https://progen.md/wp-content/uploads/2020/12/9476_covid_19_impactul_wellbeing.pdf.

DW. (2022). Moldova has reached the brink of a demographic drama. 26.01.2022. https://www.dw.com/ro/moldova-a-ajuns-%C3%AEn-pragul-unei-drame-demografice/a-60560631

Government of the Republic of Moldova. (2020). *Republic of Moldova voluntary national. review progress report* 2020

Heubeck, B., Watson, J., & Russell, R. (1986). Father involvement and responsibility in family therapy. In M. E. Lamb (Ed.), *The father's role: Applied perspectives* (pp. 191–226). Wiley.

IFIS. (2021). https://ifis.md/evenimente/grup-de-suport-pentru-femei/

NBS. (2020). https://statbank.statistica.md/PxWeb/pxweb/ro/30%20Statistica%20sociala/?rxid=b2ff27d7-0b96-43c9-934b-42e1a2a9a774

NBS. (2021). *Statistical yearbook of the Republic of Moldova*. National Bureau of Statistics of the Republic of Moldova. https://statistica.gov.md/files/files/publicatii_electronice/Anuar_Statistic/2021/Anuar_statistic_editia_2021.pdf

OSCE. (2019). OSCE-led survey on violence against women. Well-Being and safety of women. Moldova results report. https://www.osce.org/files/f/documents/2/1/424979_0.pdf

Popovici, L. (2019). Documentarea violenţei în bază de gen: Ghid practic [Documentation of gender-based violence: Practical guide]. Chişinău: S. n. (Tipogr. "Depol Promo").

UN Women. (2021). *Republic of Moldova country gender equality brief*. United Nations.

UNDP. (2020). Human development report 2020. The next frontier: Human development and the Anthropocene. *Briefing note for countries on the 2020 human development report.* .

UNFPA, MMPS. (2022). *Teoria schimbării pentru rezilienţa demografică [Theory of change for demographic Resilience]*. UNFPA, Ministry of Labour and Social Protection. https://moldova.unfpa.org/sites/default/files/pub-pdf/teoria_schimbarii_pentru_rezilienta_demografica_-_adaptare_atenuare_ajustare.pdf

Walters, J., Tasker, F., & Bichard, S. (2001). 'Too busy'? Fathers' attendance for family appointments. *Journal of Family Therapy, 23*(1), 3–20. https://doi.org/10.1111/1467-6427.00166

Chapter 6
Sociocultural Traumatization and Resilience in Serbia: Family Legacies at the Turn of the Millennium

Tamara Džamonja Ignjatović, Nevena Čalovska Hercog, Biljana Stanković, and Smiljka Tomanović

The authors of this chapter share an interest in families and the impact of social changes on their structure and dynamic; however, we approach the topic from different but complementary perspectives of sociology (ST), social and clinical psychology (TDžI & BS), and psychotherapy (NČH). It was a challenge for us to start from different scientific and practical experiences and find the common "meet point" that could contribute to improving understanding and therapeutic approach to families in the specific social, political, and cultural context of Serbia.

Overview of the Sociocultural Context of Trauma

Demographics

The Republic of Serbia is a small country in the southeast European region (see Map 4, Appendix, this volume), usually referred to as the West Balkans. As a consequence of negative population growth that started in the 1970s, the country has been facing a constant depopulation: from 7.7 million in 1994 to 6.8 million

T. D. Ignjatović (✉) · B. Stanković
University of Belgrade, Faculty of Philosophy, Department of Psychology, Belgrade, Serbia

N. Č. Hercog
University Singidunum, Faculty of Media and Communications, Department of Psychology, Belgrade, Serbia

S. Tomanović
University of Belgrade, Faculty of Philosophy, Department of Psychology, Belgrade, Serbia

University of Belgrade, Faculty of Philosophy, Department of Sociology, Belgrade, Serbia

T. Glebova, C. Knudson-Martin (eds.), *Sociocultural Trauma and Well-Being in Eastern European Family Therapy*, AFTA SpringerBriefs in Family Therapy,
https://doi.org/10.1007/978-3-031-29995-7_6

inhabitants in 2021 (Vukmirović, 2014). The death rate increased in 2020 and particularly in 2021, when there was a 26.5% increase of deaths as compared to 2020. Another source of depopulation is a huge emigration flow, particularly in the last decade (Statistical Office of the Republic of Serbia XE "Serbia", 2021). Projections indicate that the population of Serbia will decrease by around 5% by 2030, and about 15–20% by 2050, mostly due to migration of younger population (Batog et al., 2019). The result is an aging population, where citizens over 64 comprise more than one-fifth, while children under 14 comprise less than 15% of the population at the moment, with a decrease and aging of the working population, increase of the old-age dependence, and pressure on healthcare and pension systems.

Although Serbia is a secular state, only around 5% of people declare as nonreligious, while the others identify themselves as Christian, mainly Orthodox (over 80%), and around 3% as Muslim. The ethnic composition reflects the religious identification: over 80% of citizens are ethnically Serbs, with other Slavic people (Bosnians, etc.), Hungarians, and Roma comprising the remaining populations.

The World Bank classifies Serbia as a middle-income country: GDP per capita in 2020 was 6533 USD or 5440 EUR (EUROSTAT, 2022). Transition of the economy from being dominated by the state sector to a market-driven model has two major consequences: the constant increase of GDP per capita (with a decrease during the global economic crisis 2009–2015) and the constant increase of economic and social inequalities.

There is continuous, although slow, progress in improving gender equality: Gender Equality Index for the Republic of Serbia based on data from 2018 amounts to 58.0 points, which is an increase of 5.6 points as compared to 2014.[1] "If progress continues at this pace, it will take 59 years to achieve full gender equality at a high level of achievement in the domains covered by the Index" (Babović & Petrović, 2021, p. 10). Considering the Global Gender Gap Index of 0.7360, Serbia held 39th place in 2020 (Global gender gap report, 2021).

According to the latest census in 2011, there are trends of an increase in the share of single households (mainly comprised of people over 65), decrease of two-parent families' households, and a slight increase of the share of households with couples without children and of single parents with children. Serbia is characterized by a decreasing, but still relatively high, share of extended family households (Statistical Office of the Republic of Serbia Census, 2021). There are high and relatively stable marriage rates with a very low share of cohabitation, which was 8.5% in the population over 15 (ibid), and a relatively low share of divorce, at 1.60% in 2019.

[1]The Gender Equality Index is a tool to measure the progress of gender equality, developed by European Institute for Gender Equality (EIGE). It takes into consideration 31 indicators in six core domains—work, money, knowledge, time, power, and health: https://eige.europa.eu/gender-equality-index. The average score for the EU countries was 68 points in 2021, from the lowest of 52.5 points in Greece to the highest of 83.9 points in Sweden.

Historical, Political, and Economic Transitions

It is important to understand the above demographics within the context of the historical events, as well as political and economic transitions. During the twentieth century and at the beginning of the twenty-first century, a series of historical events in Serbia, as a part of the Former Yugoslavia, contributed to the specific pattern of repetitive social traumatization.

After liberation from the Ottoman Empire, during the nineteenth century, Serbia was established as a constitutional monarchy based on patriarchal values and the rural way of life. Despite the devastation of the country, World War I led to the unification of Serbia with other South Slavic nations who lived under the former Habsburg monarchy, and on December first of 1918, the new country, Yugoslavia (under the original name Kingdom of Serbs, Croats, and Slovenians) was born (compare Maps A.1 and A.2, Appendix, this volume). Characterized by significant cultural, ethnic, and religious diversities and political conflicts rooted in national antagonism, Yugoslavia was faced with the Second World War. The country was devastated again by the German occupation and at the same time by the civil conflicts between different ethnic groups. During that period, more than a hundred thousand Serbs, Jews, and Roma people were victims of a genocide committed by the Ustashe, Croatian fascist movement. The victory of the Communist Partisans resulted in the constitution of Socialist Federal Republic of Yugoslavia, a one-party state established by the Communist Party of Yugoslavia under President Tito. During that period, the country experienced industrial progress, which was strongly supported by the promotion of national brotherhood-unity and nonaligned international politics.

After the 1990s, the breakup of Yugoslavia began, based on the previous antagonisms and unfulfilled aspirations of different ethnic and religious groups, leading to the secession of former Yugoslav republics, which declared independence (see current national borders in Map 4, Appendix, this volume). Fueled by ethnic tensions, Yugoslav Wars (1991–1999) erupted, leading to brutal warfare and violence in Croatia, Bosnia, and Kosovo, where ethnic Serb communities opposed independence from Yugoslavia. The United Nations imposed sanctions against Serbia that led to political isolation, collapse of the economy, and a high record of inflation. Finally, NATO intervened by bombing Serbia and established UN administration in the province of Kosovo, while Serbia became home to a high number of refugees and internally displaced persons, mainly from Croatia, Bosnia and Herzegovina, and Kosovo. Although Serbian citizens engaged in large protests against the government throughout the decade, the regime of Milosevic resisted until 2000. Finally, on October fifth, half a million people from all over the country protested in Belgrade, compelling Milošević to concede defeat. This ended Yugoslavia's international isolation and the EU opened negotiations with the country for the Stabilization and Association Agreement.

However, Serbia's political climate remained tense, and in 2003, the Prime Minister Zoran Đinđić, who was promising for democratic changes, was assassinated. The short period of democracy, progress, and hope ended soon since the party close to the Milosevic regime won the elections in 2012. At present, Serbia suffers from democratic backsliding leading to authoritarianism, political tensions, increased corruption, social inequalities, and a decline in media freedom and civil rights. The refugee crisis in Europe also hit this region since Serbia is on the route of refugees from Syria, Afghanistan, Iraq, etc. Finally, the COVID-19 pandemic additionally burdened the country.

The multitude of historical and cultural transformations during the twentieth and the beginning of the twenty-first century, including ethnic conflicts, wars, profound social changes from rural and patriarchal society, transitions from socialism and industrialization that reflected positively on workers' rights, social security and ethnic and gender equality, to the liberal capitalism accompanied by uncertainty and social stratification, has been affecting people and their families for decades in Serbia. These dramatic changes and long-lasting crises and conflict beyond personal control leave many people feeling helpless, which becomes a fertile ground for sociocultural trauma, particularly for people from multiethnic families.

Current Sociocultural, Economic, and Political Contexts

After the period of total collapse of the economy during the 1990s, there has been economic recovery since 2000, with an increase of GDP, except during the global economic crisis. At the same time, market reforms, particularly those based on neoliberal models of development in the social context of weak institutions and a corrupted state unsupported by the rule of law, led to the sharp increases in social inequalities and number of people living in poverty (income inequality is currently the highest among European countries).

Certain anti-modern trends continue throughout post-socialist transformation. For instance, there is a widespread system of corruption in various segments of society, which is noticed by citizens and normalized by young people (Lavrič et al., 2019). During a period of nationalistic appraisal during the 1990s, but also after 2000, Serbia has witnessed strong re-traditionalization of the public discourse and sphere, including de-secularization and the rise of right-wing movements and organizations.

The existing welfare regime in Serbia can be defined as post-socialist version of a sub-protective regime (Esping-Andersen, 1996), which postulates that families provide resources for various needs of their members. Together with the unfinished economic and social system transformation, frequent global economic fluctuations, rising economic and social inequality, deinstitutionalization and political clientelism in the state systems, and low trust in corrupted institutions, it comprises the social and cultural contexts for family lives.

Findings from many studies point to a conservative view of family life dominated by familism (Tomanović, 2017), even among young people in Serbia, which is evidenced through high value placed on starting a family, marriage, and childbirth

(Popadić et al., 2019). Related to gender norms, several studies suggest the self-realization of identity through gender roles of "caring mother" for women and "responsible breadwinner" for men (Tomanović, 2021; Stanojević, 2018). During the post-socialist transformation in Serbia, the population became impoverished, which led to intensifying work and diversifying the working strategies of individuals and families, often through a combination of formal, and additional informal work. The social protection system collapsed, which resulted in a greater reliance on informal forms of family support and exchange. Intergenerational family support is crucial in early parenthood, as studies on young parents' experiences reveal (Tomanović, 2012). One-parent families, particularly single mothers, are heavily dependent on support of their parental families, but are the least likely to get it (Tomanović et al., 2014).

Families have been heavily burdened with providing material resources and caring activities to their members—children, young, and elderly (Milić et al., 2010). This also produces constant gender inequality in domestic work and caring activities. Intergenerational solidarity in both directions became particularly prominent in the context of the COVID-19 pandemic (Tomanović, 2021), as well as a specific burden on women performing caring activities (Čikić & Bilinović Rajačić, 2020). The consequences of this kind of networked family relations could be manifested as difficulties with individualization within partners' relationship and generational relations within the family (Tomanović, 2017), which is further related to frequent occurrence of family violence and conflict and ambivalence in intergenerational relations (e.g., Tomanović, 2021).

Experience of the Sociocultural and Transgenerational Trauma

As elaborated in the introduction (Glebova et al., Chap. 1, this volume), sociocultural trauma is both a clinical and a socio-psychological concept. Besides afflicting individuals, it also affects their social environment, possibly initiating long-term consequences involving families and sometimes even the whole communities (Hamburger, 2021a). The concept of sociocultural trauma calls for acknowledging the historical and sociopolitical origins and perpetuating conditions of individual and family trauma, which requires a more nuanced and broader approach than that usually adopted in psychology and psychiatry, both in research and in clinical practice. Keeping in mind the description of the local historical context given previously, it is obvious that Serbia is replete with socio-traumatic history. Its people have been repeatedly exposed to ethnic, religious, and ideological conflicts, mass forced migrations from neighboring countries and provinces, and accompanying economic, social, and political turmoil that led to prolonged existential insecurities.

What further perpetuates the situation of crisis and uncertainty and complicates the processes of stabilization and reconciliation are the dominant sociopolitical narratives that involve targeted use and biased interpretation of the past. Since the beginning of the 1990s the representations of the past historical events during which Serbian people were persecuted or victimized are revitalized and encouraged as part of the current political propaganda. As proposed by the concept of the chosen trauma, this reactivates unresolved feelings of loss and mourning, thus facilitating regression, defensive reactions, and feelings of entitlement to revenge, leading to aggressive feelings and behaviors toward out-groups recognized as historical enemies (Volkan, 2006, 2021). An especially prominent place in Serbian collective memory is given to the "Kosovo myth,"[2] which is also often recognized as Serbian chosen trauma. It became an important marker of Serbian national identity, especially after the demise of Yugoslavia, reactivated repeatedly throughout both distant and recent sociopolitical conflicts and their aftermaths.

Although the "Kosovo myth" refers to a distant historical event, its psycho-social consequences are current and far-reaching. In the everyday experiences and imaginations of the Serbian people, the national and religious conflicts are kept alive, even years or decades after their formal termination. This enables the transmission and perpetuation of social trauma in families and communities in Serbia, where complex and long-term sociohistorical processes and events, not just the recent or current ones, play a prominent role. It also emphasizes the crucial role of cultural artifacts and media representations in the processes of collective coping and traumatic healing.

The socio-traumatic consequences of these historical and sociopolitical processes are profound and long-lasting. The ones that are probably easiest to assess are those potentially affecting individuals and families directly involved in the conflicts during the most recent wars—soldiers and their families, as well as the refugees from Bosnia and Herzegovina, Croatia, and Kosovo—their numbers ranging from tens to hundreds of thousands. But there are also a number of families indirectly affected—from those providing shelter to their refugee family members and friends to all those living through the scarcities and insecurities of war times, political upheaval, and extreme economic inflation. While we should not reduce the concept of social trauma to a psychopathological category, it is possible to recognize a number of symptoms in afflicted individuals that predominantly fit into the category of posttraumatic disorders (Hamburger, 2021a), often accompanied by substance abuse, suicidal thoughts, depression, and anxiety, or anger and violence.

There is also an additional range of symptoms, including hopelessness, low self-esteem, prolonged sadness, social withdrawal, and problems of emotional regulation (Hamburger, 2021b) that lead to poor mental health and quality of life. Studies of war veterans, who find themselves in the role of perpetrator, victim, or witness at the same time, often suffer from PTSD, with the burden of guilt and shame, and turn their unbearable tension as aggressive acts toward themselves or externalize it toward others. Studies in Serbia confirmed the high risk of suicide or family

[2] Related to the events during the Battle of Kosovo in the fourteenth century, that ended in Turkish victory and collapse of Serbia, but in the collective memory of Serbs it was a glorious defeat, proof of courage, and resistance to slavery regardless of the victims.

violence among war veterans (Beara, 2011). One study (Radetić Lovrić & Pećanac, 2020) focused on the far-reaching psychological consequences of the war in the former Yugoslavia (1991–1995) and examined the relationships between wartime traumatic experience of loss, quality of life, and mental health. The results showed that respondents who continue to search for the body of a missing family member have a lower quality of life and have a more pronounced presence of depressive and psychosomatic symptoms.

There are also indicators on the social level that we might consider metaphorically as "symptoms" inflicted on the collective body, especially regarding the conspiracy of silence, erosion of institutions, hate speech (Hamburger, 2021b), and simplistic representations of the complex historical and political realities, which are all continuously present in Serbian public space. This is especially important when considering the phenomenon of the transgenerational transmission of trauma that links the individual and family level to the social environment, since the individual strategies of coping and resources for narrativization and integration of traumatic experiences and events, in cases of social trauma, are also shaped by available representations of traumatic events or unresolved conflicts on the collective level (Hamburger, 2021a), or, as is more often the case in Serbia, by the conspiracy of silence or defensive reactions.

Illustrative of the processes mentioned above are the findings of one recent qualitative research that analyzed biographical narratives of family members of different generations living in Serbia, with a focus on their experiences and representations of turning-point events in the social, individual, and family history (Đorđević et al., 2018). The aim was to explore the specificities and differences in the way relevant sociopolitical events are represented and narrated within families. The analysis pointed out significant gender and generational differences. Women belonging to the middle and the older generation (mothers and grandmothers) elaborate on events and experiences that are central to periods of intense social, political, and economic changes in Serbia, especially during the 1990s. They recognize their central role in shaping personal and family life, which is narrated through concrete, intense, and potentially traumatic experiences, described in great detail and in an emotionally involved way. In contrast, men of the middle and the older generation (fathers and grandfathers) show a common pattern of avoiding the narrativization of social events—they explicitly distance themselves from the social and political sphere and focus on personal/family experiences. Many of them were also direct participants in the political or war events (as mobilized soldiers or party members), but they show defeatism, disappointment, and a cultural "conspiracy of silence" in connection with these experiences, all of which can be an indicator of a socio-traumatic experience that is not yet integrated.

In the narratives of family members of the youngest generation (children in adolescence or emergent adulthood), regardless of gender, the description of important social events is usually missing and they are focused on individual experiences and normative developmental tasks (finishing school, getting a job, entering a serious relationship) (Đorđević et al., 2018). The family system, which protects young people from the influence of turbulent sociopolitical events, is probably partly responsible for that. Prominent lack of interest in politics and wider sociopolitical events among young people, as well as insufficient information about them, with occasional expressions of distrust in the system, skepticism, and disappointment, is supported by the fact that young people, unlike previous generations, do not have direct experience of different sociopolitical circumstances than those in which they grew up, and live in a state of "permanent crisis" to which they have become accustomed over time.

These insights indicate that both gender and generational differences significantly shape specific patterns of affectivity, narrativization of experiences, and personal relationships that are characteristic of individual family members. Additionally, neuralgic points that are surrounded by the vow of silence in family narratives suggest that the broken threads in the social narrative are reproduced at the family and individual levels.

Challenges for Family Therapy

Living in the same social context and sharing isomorphic experiences at all levels requires a family therapist to have knowledge of the effects of complex, historical, and intergenerational trauma. Socio-traumatic background leads to specific patterns and problems in the processes of parenting, attachment, and values transmission. Family therapists have a crucial role in assisting families in more successfully negotiating social change while deconstructing and reconstructing trauma-saturated narratives.

Given that the transgenerational aspect in social trauma is a unique form of traumatic exposure, therapy can be effective in reducing its negative long-term effects. There are specific components of trauma that must be addressed. Because the attachment relationship between a parent or caregiver and a child is one of the possible mechanisms through which transgenerational trauma is transmitted, treatment should focus on the important familial and interpersonal patterns relative to the client and utilize attachment-focused interventions.

Effective treatment for those experiencing trauma also focuses on exploring, developing, and maintaining protective factors that can reduce the negative impact of trauma. Some protective factors include fostering secure attachment between a parent and a child as well as having access to several sources of support (i.e., family, peers, or community). For example, "transgenerational scripts," which are unconscious systemic patterns that persist in families and groups, are perpetuated through emotions, beliefs, and behaviors. These scripts are then used to explore clients' implicit and explicit perceptions about their family dynamic and system. Therapists can guide clients to separate their ancestors' experiences from their own and help them make sense of what happened with an emphasis on building resilience.

Case Example

The following case illustrates how past experiences and present context influence the behaviors, beliefs, and values of family members and contribute to the problems and conflictual relations among them. This was an upper middle-class, urban Serbian family, living in a three-generation constellation, where the maternal grandmother is a refugee from Croatia since 2005 and a widow (husband killed as an army officer in military actions in 1995). She has been a primary caretaker to two, now adolescent, children of her daughter. Her daughter, unwillingly a housewife as she could not find employment as a sculptress, is married to a businessman. They contacted the family therapist because of many difficulties: marital distress (husband was having an extramarital "office affair"); mother was receiving outpatient medical treatment due to exacerbation of her autoimmune ophthalmological condition; an older son, seventeen years old and finishing high school stopped attending classes and was spending most of his time in his room, talking exclusively with his grandmother, playing video games; a younger sixteen-year-old son was staying out late, declining in academic results, defying both parents and grandmother, and joining a national soccer fan club with explicit right-wing political nationalistic convictions. Parents reported constantly balancing their needs to hold on to their values and scripts, especially those that were shaped by the sociopolitical context of family history and tradition. Some of these, such as "rely on your family only," "people are selfish," "world is unjust, unpredictable and dangerous," were adopted from their parents and transferred to their children, while adapting to tremendous continuous changes due to unstable political environments, dominant materialistic values, and the increasing influence of technology. This struggle seemed to cluster mainly around family togetherness versus autonomy. Parents openly spoke of their fear that their sons would break away from them and be unprepared for independent life and get hurt from the "outside world."

The need to balance different values, especially those that are socio-traumatically shaped, was the most significant experience in negotiating differences between the generations. In order to keep their influence on their children despite social changes, the parents needed to change their transfer strategies, which were discussed and dealt with in therapy sessions. Family routines were structured to be "time and space" for reflecting, not instructing. This priority of keeping a warm relationship was found to facilitate some value transmission between the parents and their sons by making them eager to be similar to the parents and to please them. Instead of using didactic methods such as warning or telling how to behave, they used modeling and routines, such as family dinners and nonintrusive ways such as text-messaging to create an environment for their sons to enjoy family togetherness and internalize it. Instead of having the last word as their parents had, they have negotiated to find the middle ground and become satisfied with partial compliance to balance the relationship with autonomy.

However, these parents remained very concerned regarding their sons. Their concerns can be understood as the lingering effect of sociocultural trauma. Traumatic and violent death of the grandfather, both implicitly and explicitly, generates ongoing parental worrying, which very well accommodates traditional Serbian stereotypical parental roles as well. Since they realized that they could not physically constrain them, they tried to be close to them so as to learn what they were exposed to from their peers and the media. By being open with each other and increasingly involved in their schoolwork and social life, they felt that they had a chance to keep an eye on them. Thus, although the hierarchical control was diminished, a protective and nurturing control was initiated reflecting a heightened worry about children's safety because of the past experience (loss of grandfather in the war) as well as persistent social turbulence, conflict, and uncertainty.

Although these parents had some differences in the beginning, they affected each other's values with time and achieved a synthesis. They were seen separately by the therapist as a parental subsystem. As they insisted that family should have meals together, they were able to break the social conspiracy of silence and keep themes they experienced in their family of origin by telling stories from their past, remembering feelings and family decisions shaped by different social events. Although the mother and the father mostly agreed on their core values, there were some significant differences between their experiences of value transmission. Mother was more concerned with what they could not transfer to their children, questioned their parenting, and looked for confirmation from others. On the other hand, father normalized their parenting and children's differences, acknowledging generational norms. In the end, the father emphasized the result, whereas the mother was concerned with the process. Both of them felt they were unable to transmit the most important values to their children exactly as they internalized them in their families of origin but tried to negotiate the content of those values with their sons. Therapy provided context for voicing generational and gender differences and giving the family permission to openly discuss and negotiate differences across time.

Implications for Clinical Practice

In conceptualizing treatment, it is critical to take into account the ways in which various cultural and sociopolitical factors impact how treatment may be received or perceived. Although the mechanisms through which transgenerational trauma is transmitted are consistent across cultures, there are variations in the degree of salience regarding sociocultural factors that may exacerbate the effects of trauma in different marginalized communities. Additionally, therapists must incorporate a culturally responsive perspective. It is imperative to focus on establishing a concrete basis of trust and safety within the therapeutic relationship, as traumatized clients may have developed significant mistrust within interpersonal interactions, as well as mistrust of larger organizations or institutions.

Rapid and drastic change in societal norms, namely from patriarchal and socialist to western, created an intergenerational clash of cultures within families. Parents find themselves facing daily decisions about prioritizing familial values and allowing their adolescents to be influenced by the new hybrid culture. In addition to normative intergenerational tensions ("generation gap"), essentially burdened and shaped by living in a context that is continuously socio-traumatically affected, they experience an internal struggle between freedom and dependence, separateness and togetherness, and nurturing and autonomy. These dilemmas may create confusion and a sense of powerlessness for parents who may resist adapting to the new generation's negative feedback, which may escalate intergenerational or even parental conflict. On the other hand, these dilemmas have the potential to create a constructive tension that may result in a new synthesis. Family therapists have a crucial role in assisting people in more successfully negotiating social change while deconstructing and reconstructing trauma-saturated narratives.

While exploring origins of scripts of trauma and survival and their relevance to a current societal context, therapists need to assist parents to find ways that will satisfy each member in the family. While balancing this bidirectionality, sometimes parents feel they have become too child-focused and have lost their authority status and boundaries. Often, trying to ensure that their children do not experience traumatic growing up as they did, they end up undertaking children's responsibilities such as schoolwork, arrange their lives around children's schedules, and provide them with anything they want. This invites the children to become irresponsible, self-centered, materialistic, and careless for social issues and leads them to possibly become unsatisfied adults. Parents need help opening space for the adolescent's changing values and life choices but still maintaining their boundaries. When a teen is brought to therapy for being irresponsible and only caring for himself, the therapist may encourage the parents to look at whether their parenting strategies support what they expect from the teen. For parents, it is highly insightful to track the emergence and maintenance of "overprotection" of their children as a posttraumatic strategy.

Therapists are aware that some values in families are transferred less consciously. Some value gaps may result in unintentional polarization within the family relationship (traditional vs. modern, collectivistic vs. individualistic, religious vs. atheistic, nationalistic and ethnocentric vs. internationalistic and ethno-relativistic, "Europeistic"/pro-Europe vs. "pro-Russian" orientation, etc.). The therapist needs to understand how people change as a result of sociopolitical developments in their environments and talk about this with families in a safe therapeutic environment.

Therapists must also be aware of their own values as an important component in the family's ecosystem. Being a part of the same ecosystem and sharing common experiences puts specific demands on the therapist's position. In a deeply divided and conflicted society, situations where families or some of their members have different political values compared to the therapist's can be challenging. It is of paramount importance for therapists to maintain supervision of their work and to be aware of and distinguish their political and therapeutic actions. This is additionally complex as family therapists are, and should be, trained to be socially responsible and culturally sensitive.

Conclusion

There are a lot of reasons to speak of the continuous social trauma that has been going on in Serbia in the last several decades, encompassing simple, complex, historical, and intergenerational traumas. Speaking in terms of the Olson's three-dimension model of family functioning—adaptability, cohesion, and communication (Olson et al., 1979), we could say that Serbian families are facing a prolonged demand to adapt to traumatic circumstances, where some "deviant" adaptation could be considered "a normal response to the abnormal reality." Threatening circumstances are challenging for family cohesion, too, whether it contributes to weakening cohesion and increase of egocentricity and alienation or to strengthening symbiotic relations among family members.

Finally, social and family relations are prone to be modeled by the public discourse, supported by the media, which promotes conflict, competitive, aggressive, and often violent communication, where mistrust and intolerance prevail. Besides symptoms of posttraumatic disorders, experiences of hopelessness, sadness, anxiety, anger, and violence, the consequences of collective traumatic experiences lead to chronic vulnerability for re-traumatization in facing upcoming threatening events. It is also important to bear in mind that people developed resilience toward new stressors and traumas. The results of a recent qualitative study confirmed that resilient individuals have developed some protective internal coping mechanisms as "a philosophy of acceptance"; they have already survived various bad things and realize "that just happens in life, too, and ends once, sooner or later" (Džamonja Ignjatović et al., 2020, p. 216). The same study also confirmed that social relations and emotional support of close and important others play the main protective role. Therefore, family therapists should enhance a sense of closeness and togetherness, as one of the most important factors of resilience. Instead of silence and withdrawal, which is typical for traumatic reactions in order to spare others from facing difficult feelings, therapists should support family members to understand and openly talk about traumatic damage, nurturing close relations as the essence of successful family therapy and process of trauma healing. Doing so requires that therapists develop a high level of personal tolerance to uncertainty and instability, focusing on finding sources of resilience and meaning in life.

***

While we were writing this chapter, the war in Ukraine started. This recent war in the neighborhood is a new, twofold, challenge for people and families in Serbia. Past traumatic experiences are still latently present, not just in memory, but also as an unresolved ethnic and political tension that could be easily reignited. Fear that the conflict may spread to our area and that such experiences may be repeated is potentially re-traumatizing. When looking at what the people in Ukraine are going through, with deep empathy for victims and their losses, images of destruction and refugees from personal experience inevitably emerge for many. On the other hand, the escalation of negative counter-reactions to the Russian people also triggers memories of the past. Russian people suffer from the consequences of their totalitarian regime, too. Exclusion of their artists, scientists, and athletes from concerts, competitions, or memberships of different organizations, expatriation of Russians living in foreign countries who left Russia because they didn't want to live under such regime, left them with a feeling that they do not belong anywhere. That "conflicting role" of being perceived solely as a persecutor and at the same time feeling as a victim, without the possibility to control personal life and choices, without a "right place to stand," is the experience close to many people from Serbia.

Every injustice has its prehistory and represents a reaction to a previous one, and at the same time, it leads to new future injustices in which everyone becomes a potential victim, thus creating conditions for the constant recurrence of transgeneration trauma in individuals and families in Serbia or any other conflicted part of the world.

References

Babović, M., & Petrović, M. (2021). *Gender equality index for the Republic of Serbia 2021*. Social inclusion and poverty reduction unit of the government of the Republic of Serbia.

Batog, C., Crivelli, E., Ilyina, A., Jakab, Z., Lee, J., Musayev, A., Petrova, I., Scott, A., Shabunina, A., Tudyka, A., Xu, X. C., & Zhang, R. (2019). *Demographic headwinds in central and Eastern Europe, European departmental paper series, no. 19*. International Monetary Fund, European Department.

Beara, V. (2011). War veterans and family violence. In D. J. Christie (Ed.), *The encyclopedia of peace psychology*. Blackwell Publishing.

Čikić, J., & Bilinović Rajačić, A. (2020). Family practices during the pandemic and the state of emergency. *Sociološki pregled, 54*(3), 799–836.

Đorđević, A., Stanković, B., Grbić, S., & Ristić, S. (2018). Narrativization of social events in the family: Analysis of turning-point events in family members of three generations. In V. Džinović i S. Grbić (Ed.), *Kvalitativna istraživanja u društvenim naukama: Od ličnog iskustva do socijalnih praksi* (pp. 97–101). IPI & Filozofski fakultet u Beogradu.

Džamonja Ignjatović, T., Stanković, B., & Klikovac, T. (2020). Experiences and quality of life of the elderly during the Covid19 pandemic and the introduction of restrictive measures in Serbia. *Psihološka istraživanja, 23*(2), 201–231.

Esping-Andersen, G. (1996). *Welfare States in Transition: National Adaptations in Global Economies*. Sage.

EUROSTAT. (2022). https://ec.europa.eu/eurostat/statisticsexplained/index.php? title=Enlargement_countries_-_statistical_overview. Retrieved on 16 June 2022.

Global Gender Gap Report. (2021). https://www.weforum.org/reports/global-gender-gap-report-2021/. Retrieved on 16 June 2022.

Hamburger, A. (2021a). Social trauma: A bridging concept. In A. Hamburger, C. Hancheva, & V. Volkan (Eds.), *Social trauma. An interdisciplinary textbook (pp. 3–15)*. Springer.

Hamburger, A. (2021b). The complexity of social trauma diagnosis and intervention. In A. Hamburger, C. Hancheva, & V. Volkan (Eds.), *Social trauma. An interdisciplinary textbook (pp. 3–15)*. Springer.

Lavrič, M., Tomanović, S., & Jusić, M. (2019). *Youth study Southeast Europe 2018/2019*. Friedrich Ebert Stiftung.

Milić, A., Tomanović, S., Ljubičić, M., Sekulić, N., Bobić, M., Miletić-Stepanović, V., & Stanojević, D. (2010). Family times. In *Sociological study on family transformation in contemporary Serbia*. Belgrade: Institute for Sociological Research.

Olson, D., Sprenkle, D., & Russell, C. (1979). Circumplex model of marital and family systems: I. cohesion and adaptability dimensions, family types, and clinical application. *Family Process, 18*(1), 3–18.
Popadić, D., Pavlović, Z., & Mihailović, S. (2019). *Youth study Serbia 2018/2019*. Friedrich Ebert Stiftung.
Radetić Lovrić, S., & Pećanac, A. (2020). Quality of life after traumatic loss and the role of social support: Examining the psychological consequences of the war twenty-five years later. *Psihološka Istraživanja, 23*(2), 121–140.
Stanojević, D. (2018). *New fatherhood in Serbia: A sociological study of practices and identities of fathers*. Belgrade: Institute for Sociological Research.
Statistical Office of the Republic of Serbia. (2021). https://www.stat.gov.rs/enus/oblasti/stanovnistvo/ procene-stanovnistva/. Retrieved on 16 June 2022.
Tomanović, S. (2012). Family transitions. In S. Tomanović, D. Stanojević, I. Jarić, D. Mojić, S. Dragišić Labaš, & M. Ljubičić (Eds.), *Young people are present. Study of social biographies of young people in Serbia* (pp. 127–147). Belgrade: Institute for Sociological Research.
Tomanović, S. (2017). Parenthood between familism and individualisation: The case of Serbia. In S. Ignjatović & A. Bošković (Eds.), *Individualism* (pp. *162–181*) Belgrade: Institute for Social Sciences.
Tomanović, S. (2021). Family practices and solidarity during COVID-19 pandemic in Serbia. Qualitative analysis of "family stories". In M. Petrović (Ed.), *Challenges in the sphere of work, family life and lifestyle in COVID-19 context in Serbia* (pp. *65–80*). Belgrade: Faculty of Philosophy.
Tomanović, S., Ljubičić, M., & Stanojević, D. (2014). *Jednoroditeljske porodice u Srbiji – sociološka studija (One-parent Families in Serbia – Sociological Study)*. Belgrade: Čigoja & Institute for Sociological Research.
Volkan, V. D. (2006). *Killing in the name of identity: A study of bloody conflicts*. Pitchstone Publishing.
Volkan, V. D. (2021). Chosen traumas and their impact on current political/societal conflicts. In A. Hamburger, C. Hancheva, & V. Volkan (Eds.), *Social trauma. An interdisciplinary textbook (pp. 17–24)*. Springer.
Vukmirović, D. (2014). *Comparative overview of the number of population 1948, 1953, 1961, 1971, 1981, 1991, 2002 and 2011*. Statistical Office of the Republic of Serbia.

Chapter 7
Sociocultural Trauma and Intergenerational Relational Ethics

Tatiana Glebova and Carmen Knudson-Martin

Long before I (Tatiana) decided to become a family therapist and began to study its major models, I was puzzled by seeing that some people who went through a lot of suffering themselves lacked sympathy toward others going through similar ordeals. I thought one's own experience of pain and struggle would make it easier to empathize with the pain of others, but often witnessed the opposite. In contextual therapy, I found an explanation in the phenomenon called destructive entitlement. The theory and the clinical model of Ivan Boszormenyi-Nagy's contextual therapy resonated with my personal background and worldview. As a researcher and clinician, it is important to me that contextual theory has a strong explanatory power to understand many dynamics of human relationships, and its clinical approach focuses on human connections and relational fairness as a foundation and resource for our lives, both as individuals and members of a larger society. Thus, our interconnectedness and its unavoidable ethical consequences are central to the model.

I (Carmen) was also drawn to contextual therapy's emphasis on the ethical nature of our relationships with one another. It is the only clinical model that I am aware of that puts our responsibility to others at the core and emphasizes the consequences of our clinical work on others and on the next generation. Like Tatiana, I found that contextual therapy concepts provided an answer to why some participants in my qualitative research transformed destructive patterns from the past into positive commitment to the future (Knudson-Martin, 1992). And, I was struck that while recognizing the harm or disservice done to them by their parents, they could also acknowledge the injustices their parents experienced and credit them for some

T. Glebova (✉)
Alliant International University, Sacramento, CA, USA
e-mail: tglebova@alliant.edu

C. Knudson-Martin
Emerita, Lewis & Clark College, Portland, OR, USA

T. Glebova, C. Knudson-Martin (eds.), *Sociocultural Trauma and Well-Being in Eastern European Family Therapy*, AFTA SpringerBriefs in Family Therapy,
https://doi.org/10.1007/978-3-031-29995-7_7

positive contributions to their lives. They could not escape their fundamental connection to the past, but they could be accountable for their impact on the future.

In the previous chapters, clinicians and researchers from five Eastern European countries reflected on their country's experience of sociocultural trauma and its various impacts on interpersonal and family relationships. The chapters show that while the region shares the same major historical events, each country and even groups within the same country have their own "marking events" that can be considered sources of sociocultural traumas for that particular culture. At the same time, all experienced wars, ethnic conflicts, totalitarian regimes, drastic changes of social structures, and economic hardships caused by those historical events. One overarching fact in the historical background of the countries is the intensity and high frequency of various social disturbances within a relatively short historical period that in "family time" spread across several generations. For example, in Hungary, political power changed nine times between 1918 and 1990. In addition to the state transformations of the 1990s, Moldova, Russia, and Serbia had internal war or conflicts. With those repeated, prolonged, and complex disruptions of the social environment, it is not surprising that fundamental perceptions of the world and human relations in that world have been shaken and changed. As a consequence, basic trust in human relationships is decreased, and this impact can be transmitted to future generations.

Trust and the Ethical Nature of Interconnectedness

The paramount importance of relational trust has been acknowledged by clinicians and scholars in various fields. From the sociological perspective, trust is a fundamental component of human actions and social relationships (Sztompka, 2000). Pragmatically put, trust is "a simplifying strategy" (Sztompka, 2000, p. 25) that enables one to function in complex social environments. In a relatively safe and stable environment, we constantly put trust in others to follow some rules in all daily activities, for example, when we walk in the neighborhood or drive on the highway. The situation becomes very different when the social environment is dangerous and unpredictable, and actions of "others" (defined broadly) can hurt you or your loved ones. Yet trust is foundational to human connections and crucial to "dealing with an uncertain and uncontrollable future" (Sztompka, 2000, p. 25).

The critical importance of trust has been highlighted not only for interpersonal relationships but also for social-cognitive processes and sociocultural learning. Originally a philosophical construct, epistemic trust—openness to receiving communicated information that is personally relevant and of generalizable significance, has been applied to human development and the treatment of mental and emotional functioning. Fonagy and colleagues (e.g., Fonagy & Allison, 2014) argued that complex trauma undermines the individual's capacity to learn from the social environment, taking in new information about the world from other people. Development of such trust is not limited to primary attachment processes but also includes the broader sociocultural context and can be modified through life experience.

Though it is difficult, if even possible, to count all nuances of the impact of sociocultural context on child development and caregiver(s) interactions, at least two aspects can be highlighted. First is the quality of parent–child interactions. If caregivers are constantly focused on basic survival during wars or overwhelmed by prolonged social challenges such as poverty or oppression, or feel scared, depressed, or anxious because the world around is dangerous or they lost their loved ones or their support system, they are mentally less available for their children and their responses to their children are likely to be less "child attuned." Second are the societal and cultural norms transmitted. The perfectly child-attuned caregiver may transmit, either explicitly by rules or implicitly by actions and reactions, that nobody beyond the family or even the caregiver–child dyad can be trusted. The larger social and political system may encourage either trusting or mistrusting. As described in Chap. 6 (Ignjatović et al., this volume), in Serbia the social narrative is reproduced at the family and individual level as "rely on your family only," "people are selfish," and "the world is unjust, unpredictable, and dangerous."

Trust is inevitably related to the trustworthiness of "the other," whether in social or interpersonal realms. It would be damaging to keep trusting someone who hurts or fools you. Expectations of reciprocity in human relationships are also related to the sense of relational fairness or justice, and the notion that the world is fundamentally just is an essential aspect of being a social creature (Lind, 2019). Though what is considered fair or unfair in any given situation depends on many factors, including sociocultural norms and the environment, fairness seems to be an inseparable element of human interconnectedness across cultures. Relationships with each other and the larger social world are ethical in nature. Sociocultural trauma, particularly human-imposed trauma, is always a manifestation of injustice that damages trustworthy relationships among people. The critical importance of relational trust, trustworthiness, and fairness and transgenerational consequences of their violations were highlighted in Ivan Boszormenyi-Nagy's contextual therapy model more than half a century ago.

Contextual Therapy's Intergenerational Focus

Boszormenyi-Nagy's contextual therapy is an integrative approach (e.g., Boszormenyi-Nagy & Sparks, 1984/2013; Boszormenyi-Nagy & Krasner, 1986/2014) that offers an explanatory and clinically valuable framework to address the intergenerational transmission of sociocultural trauma. The model's main assumption is our existential interdependence, our interconnectedness as a fundamental aspect of being. Probably no one, at least in the mental health field, will argue with the idea that an individual's self develops and evolves within the context of relationships. Any family systems thinker or practitioner presupposes that actions of family members impact each other. Boszormenyi-Nagy took a closer look at the dynamics of those impacts or consequences. “Life is a chain of interlocking consequences linked to the interdependence of the parent and child generations” (Boszormenyi-Nagy & Krasner, 1986/2014, p. 420). According to contextual theory, relational ethics is not a set of societal or cultural norms of morality but the fundamental nature of interconnectedness through a mutual process of giving and receiving care, to which all are innately entitled.

The contextual model stresses the importance of transgenerational processes in understanding individual and relational functioning and well-being. Boszormenyi-Nagy (Boszormenyi-Nagy & Krasner, 1986/2014) wrote, “… an ethical ledger of rights and obligations exists between a person and the human order. The context of the human order of justice and transgenerational solidarity is a silent partner to intergenerational relationships” (p. 98). Responsibility for the future generations, both of own family and posterity as a whole, is a primary ethical concern; “Making the world safe for survival is the very least that one generation owes to others” (Boszormenyi-Nagy & Krasner, 1986/2014, p. 132).

Each person or family is a link that transmits or modifies transgenerational legacy-bound messages between the past, with its inherited culture and family history, and the future. As we write this chapter in October 2022, many people in Russia face tough decisions because of Russia’s war in Ukraine and the harsh political climate—whether to protest the war or go along with it, whether to stay in the country or leave it, and so on. They ask the same question, “What will I tell my children (even unborn ones)?” While their answers vary considerably, depending on individual predispositions as well as meanings and beliefs associated with a particular event at intrapersonal, familial, and group levels, their decisions inevitably have interpersonal consequences for generations.

Totalitarianism and Hardship as Relational Context

The contextual model sees an individual with their unique qualities and personal accountability as not just a “unit of the system” but as a significant player in developmental and relational dynamics. At the same time, individuals are affected by their environment, culture, and historical time. As a Russian-speaking poet Alexander Kushner wrote in 1978, during the Soviet times, about the epoch’s impact on the individual:

> Time is skin, and not attire.
> Everlasting are its stains.
> From our own marks and etchings
> One the age’s faithful sketches
> Can like fingerprints obtain.

Among the significant sociohistorical events in the five countries in this book is a period of communist government whose duration and intensity differed for each country. Russia has a special position in the group. It was the epicenter of that social transformation and had the longest history of a totalitarian regime. It was also an oppressive power in the rest of the Eastern European block. Cherepanov (2021) provided an in-depth interdisciplinary summary and analysis of the impact of totalitarian regimes on people and their transgenerational legacies, with a particular focus on the Russian experience. To maintain control of public and private life of their citizens, the totalitarian states use many strategies, both hard and soft powers, such as mass repressions, surveillance through secret police and informants, informational control, propaganda, fearmongering, and collective responsibility promotion. While communist regimes in most of these countries transformed through the years from a harsh to a softer version of totalitarianism, state power was still controlling their citizens.

Decades of those sociopolitical practices eventually impact people's social behaviors, intrapsychic processes, and worldviews and modify culture. "Living in the upside-down world, where emotional closeness, core human values, and loyalty put people at risk and moral concessions increase the chances of survival, leaves a profound and long-term impact on the psyche of survivors and their descendants" (Cherepanov, 2021, p. 56), which she compared to "the inner world of an individual with borderline personality" (p. 57). Cherepanov described common transgenerational survival messages in the totalitarian society—"Don't hope! Don't trust! Don't show your fears and pain! Don't ask for help and don't beg for mercy!" (pp. 138–140). In this book's chapters, especially the ones on Hungary (Tarján et al., this volume, Chap. 2) and Russia (Miskova, this volume, Chap. 3), we can see how some of those culturally transmitted beliefs manifest in people's lives and in therapy, along with surviving economic hardship during wars, communist times, and more recently during a rough transition to a free-market economy. Clinicians can immediately see how these beliefs and experiences stand in the way of the foundational principles or assumptions of successful therapy—hope, trusting relationships, and vulnerability in asking for help and opening up.

Sociocultural Trauma Through the Contextual Model

Van der Meiden (2019) offered a metaphor for intergenerational connections from the contextual point of view, "Thus, giving and receiving through generations can be compared with roof tile construction; each roof tile lies partly over the previous one" (p. 59). And when there are cracks in connections between those tiles, meaning, in contextual terms, violations of fairness in care and trust between family members, future generations bear the consequences. In the event of sociocultural trauma, cracks are caused by social earthquakes.

Boszormenyi-Nagy noted that transgenerational consequences of injustice are determined not only by intrafamilial dynamics (retributive injustice) but also by "factual circumstances" (distributive injustice) (Boszormenyi-Nagy & Krasner, 1986/2014) such as belonging to a particular social group, migration, genocide, and other events that cause sociocultural trauma. At least three generations are impacted, and their relational dynamics require clinical attention. The process is not always, if ever, a linear one, such as a direct transmission of posttraumatic symptoms from parents to children, but a complex interconnected pattern of manifestations of legacies, loyalty, entitlement, and parentification issues, with each generation dealing with trauma and its effects in its own way.

Let's consider Sonja's case. Sonja (the name and some personal details are changed), a Russian-speaking immigrant to the USA, sought individual therapy for her depression and relational problems with her mother and husband. She felt unloved, especially by her mother, and recalled numerous episodes when her mother was dismissive of her needs and not caring, which still caused her a lot of pain, resentment, and anger. Sonja's mom lost her parents at the age of four during the Great Purge. While initially one of her aunts took her in, she was soon separated from her family and experienced a lot of traumatic events during WWII, which meant her mom was probably depressed for years too.

Destructive Entitlement

Sonja's mother belonged to a "survivor" generation that experienced severe direct impact of persecution and war. She went through acute trauma and immediate response to trauma and losses such as grief, depression, fear of further loss, and finding ways to survive. During the in-depth genogram exploration, Sonja understood her mother's coldness as consequences of sociohistorical circumstances of her life. As a child, she not only lost her parents, but their fate was kept secret because they were not "heroes" but "enemies of the people," and she was told that she could not talk or grieve about them. Thus, she developed destructive entitlement, the contextual therapy construct describing "... the predicament of people who have been the victim of injustices that were not repaired by the wrongdoers and of injustices that were the simple result of unfortunate circumstances" (Ducommun-Nagy, 2018, p. 3).

This distributive injustice as the result of social traumas morphed into retributive injustice in how she related to her daughter. Thus, when Sonja came to her mother with her troubles, they were dismissed as "nothing important" or she was blamed for burdening her mom. At the same time, Sonja's parents were telling her that it was dangerous to share anything about herself or her family outside the family. Sonja learned that nobody cared about her or could be trusted. In this way, a legacy of family survivorship of wars, persecution, or economic hardship perpetuated destructive entitlement for future generations.

Destructive entitlement can manifest in wounding actions toward self or others. Studies in Serbia (Ignjatović et al., this volume, Chap. 6) confirmed the high risk of suicide or family violence among war veterans. In Moldova (Bodrug-Lungu, this volume, Chap. 5), the country experiencing severe economic hardship and ongoing military tension in the Transnistria region, domestic violence is a critical societal and relational issue. Domestic violence, fueled by power given by society to a parent or to a man to use physical force to control family members, is also a manifestation of destructive entitlement that, if not interrupted, might bring about destructive consequences for children.

Loyalty

Violations of trust and fairness in the parent–child relationship, whether due to social circumstances or internal family dynamics, can lead to struggle in the expression of loyalty of which people are often unaware. Loyalty refers to a deep sense of existential commitment between people related to each other either biologically (parents, siblings, etc.) or through a mutually caring relationship (partners or peers). In the germinal book on family loyalties, Boszormenyi-Nagy wrote,

Loyalty commitments are like invisible but strong fibers which hold together complex pieces of relationship "behavior" in families as well as in larger society. To understand the functions of a group of peoples, nothing is more critical than to know who are bound together in loyalty and what loyalty means for them. (Boszormenyi-Nagy & Spark, 1984/2013, p. 39)

At the individual level, loyalty is an attitude that includes identification with the group and commitment to the group. Within the family, the fundamental essence of loyalty is to maintain the family itself. We are bound by filial loyalty (i.e., loyalty toward parents and/or caregivers) even if we do not realize it. Family loyalty commitments exist in "vertical" relationships (between generations, for example, between parents and children) and in "horizontal" ones (between siblings, intimate partners, peers). Loyalty between parent and child includes parental accountability (i.e., what parents/caregivers are expected to do to nurture their children) and filial indebtedness (i.e., the indebtedness children feel toward their parents/caregivers for the care received). The Hungarian chapter (Tarján et al., this volume, Chap. 2) offers clinical illustrations of loyalty manifestations in the second and third generations of families impacted by political prosecutions and violence. In the Serbian family's case, we can see how parental loyalties to their own parents play a significant role in an intergenerational conflict of values with their adolescent children (Ignjatović et al., this volume, Chap. 6).

Parent–Child Relations

Filial loyalty and existential debt to parents make children vulnerable to destructive parentification, a reversal of the giving-receiving process between parents and children. Destructive parentification is different from what is sometimes called instrumental parentification that may be needed for a family system in crisis, such as situations of wars or hardship when older children take adult roles of caring for family members or supporting family through work. Experience of helping adults and family may contribute to developing strengths and a sense of self-competence that may be a great resource for the future. It may have unhealthy consequences, though, if other aspects of relational ethics are damaged, for example, when parentification is prolonged and the child's contributions to the family are unacknowledged. This is what happened with little Sonja. She tried her best to care about her mom. Sonja remembered that during her childhood she tried to cheer up her mother who rarely smiled and looked sorrowful. These naïve attempts were not appreciated; on the contrary, they were perceived as foolish and annoying.

Parentification may take many forms and be transmitted through generations. Sonja was the second generation of "survivors." Her own parenting style was characterized by coldness similar to her mother's, which could be a manifestation of invisible loyalty—an indirect and problematic manifestation of loyalty when its direct expression is blocked. At the same time, it was a clear embodiment of destructive entitlement. In one of our sessions, we explored how Sonja's childhood was impacting her current relationships including the one with her adolescent son who was starting to show depressive symptoms. Sonja was able to see a transgenerational pattern, but her concern about her child was blocked by unfairness that happened to her—"but what about me?" Her legitimate right to seek justice for her destructive parentification led to misplaced compensation by her child, which is unfair and destructive for the child.

Somewhat paradoxically, destructive parentification may also manifest in an opposite parenting style—overprotection and "infantilization." This is described in the Serbian case (Ignjatović et al., Chap. 6, this volume). The parents, who experienced first-hand turmoil of drastic social changes and war-related trauma, try to protect their sons from any stress, including those developmentally and environmentally appropriate such as completion of their schoolwork. Here, the need to overprotect is not founded in problems related to the child's growth; it is a consequence of parental trauma.

Responsible Parenting

In the contextual model, "Adequate or responsible parenting is the chief dynamic principle in the intergenerational order of being" (Boszormenyi-Nagy & Krasner, 1986/2014, p. 99). Parents who have been affected by mass trauma may convey an increased emotional vulnerability to their children, and their children may in turn feel a greater sense of responsibility to take care of their parents. Survivors of mass trauma may also experience the world as a dangerous place and therefore may be over-protective toward their children. Traumatic experiences can also cause parents to display intense emotions and be less emotionally available for their children, leading to child abuse and neglect or, in other words, to practice a rejecting parenting style (Field et al., 2013). Women with PTSD have been found to engage in hostile behavior as well as physical and psychological aggression (Lang & Gartstein, 2018).

While in an insecure world due to either social violence or oppression, these practices and relationships may be adaptive, their consequences have lasting transgenerational effects. When the social environment changes because of a major social shift within their country such as rapid westernization, or by emigration, these adaptations may be perceived as maladaptive or even destructive. Sonja's son was growing up in the USA with a dominant culture of individualism and authoritative parenting that values self and respectful and close relationships between children and parents, a contrast with the parenting Sonja had in her family.

Relational Resources and Resilience

So far, we mostly focused on risk and stress factors associated with the experience of trauma by parents. This focus may lead to a damage-centered (Tuck, 2009), deficit-focused, pathologizing, and victimizing view. Avoiding this is crucial. Response to sociocultural trauma may produce not only destructive or negative effects but evoke new ways of adaptation, stimulate strengths, and create new meanings. Acknowledgement of these responses to trauma is reflected in concepts of resilience (Walsh, 2003, 2016), posttraumatic growth (Tedeschi & Calhoun, 2004), and adversity-activated development (Papadopoulos, 2007). A meta-analysis of studies of trauma transmission in the second-generation and third-generation offspring of Holocaust survivors (Sagi-Schwartz et al., 2008) found "a remarkable resilience of traumatized survivors in their parental roles, even when they personally may be traumatized profoundly" (p. 118). They identified protective factors such as prewar stable family relationships, postwar social support structures, and public commemoration.

Spontaneous or "professionally-assisted" recovering from sociocultural trauma consequences happens in the larger social context, which varies on the degree of the safety-danger dimension of the social environment. In Sonja's case, she and her family lived in a relatively safe and stable environment. The situation and help needed are different when social turmoil continues. The previous generations' messages such as "the future is unpredictable" and "anything (meaning anything bad) may happen" are confirmed and activate other survival strategies like "don't trust (anybody and the world)". While therapists cannot change the social environment, at least immediately or directly, they may strengthen the relational "immune system" (Ducommun-Nagy, 2021), or in other words protective factors—fair and trustworthy relationships among family members.

Implications for Clinical Practice

The practice of contextual therapy integrates a multidimensional theoretical conceptualization that considers and operates in the complex space of facts, individual psychology, and transactional dynamics under the umbrella of relational ethics

(Boszormenyi Nagy & Krsner, 1986/2014). Because the relational context of interdependence is the foundation of health, therapeutic interventions take into consideration not only those who are present in therapy but the entire family, at least three generations.

Contextual therapists strive to be accountable to everybody who may be potentially affected by therapeutic interventions, especially future generations. This is achieved through multidirected partiality, the principal and unique method of contextual therapy. It requires the therapist to see a situation from the perspectives of each of the individuals who are likely to be affected by the course of therapy and to give each family member a chance to present their side. For this, the therapist cannot adopt a neutral position. The therapist needs to balance their partiality by "lending weight" to those who need it most at the given moment, for example, children or family members whose suffering led to destructive entitlement. Multidirected partiality is applicable to various forms of therapy—individual, couple, or family.

Contextual therapy focuses on identifying family strengths and existing relational resources such as residual trustworthiness (Boszormenyi-Nagy & Krasner, 1986/2014, p. 64). Contextual therapists assume that people care (or have a need to care) about others and do their best under the circumstances, which is grounds for a very concrete sense of hope. The therapist's active search and support for the development of new, fair connections transmit this sense of hope, which is an essential component of therapy. In contextual terms, it is called rejunction, "a reconnection with resources from the past which can be oriented to the future with posterity in mind" (Boszormenyi-Nagy & Krasner, 1986/2014, pp. 300–301). "Techniques" seem to be simple, basic therapeutic techniques of active listening, asking questions, and "planting seeds." At the same time, any instrumental technique, such as a genogram, thought analysis, or empty chair, can be used to promote relational ethics.

Sonja was a "direct" client. So, the initial focus, which can be called "empathic partiality," was on her suffering. Acknowledgment of her past and current pains was the first step. Another focus was on acknowledgment of her attempts to care for her mother. When she talked about her childhood, the therapist responded, "when you were making funny jokes, you were showing your care for your mom, but it was ignored, ridiculed, or even punished. Probably you felt confused and hurt, and maybe powerless and worthless … and you became afraid to show your care, at least openly." It took some time to process Sonja's injury to facilitate a consideration of how now, as an adult, she can show her care toward her child and mother.

Activation of "unutilized inclinations to give" (Boszormenyi-Nagy & Krasner, 1986/2014, p. 308) among the family members is a critical "mechanism" of restoring relational trust and earning individual's constructive entitlement, the contextual therapy's term to describe the process of getting self-gains (an increase in self-worth and self-esteem) through generosity to others regardless of the response of the beneficiary—"The self benefits from due caring offered to the other" (Boszormenyi-Nagy & Krasner, 1986/2014, p. 61). While we can't change the past (broken trust and a lack of care you were entitled to), trust and entitlement can be earned. This requires action and assuming responsibility for those actions, which increase an individual's agency, autonomy, and freedom.

For Sonja, those actions were toward her mom and her child. "Some of therapy's most powerful leverages issue from the dynamic resources that exist between and across the generations" (Boszormenyi-Nagy & Krasner, 1986/2014, p. 320). An important theme of therapy was an exploration of how Sonja, remembering her past experience, might acknowledge her child's inclination to support and unburden her. Crediting, "... a recognition of people's genuine efforts at fair exchange.", (Boszormenyi-Nagy & Krasner, 1986/2014, p. 309) is facilitated by the therapeutic process, but it is up to family members to define what that fair exchange is.

While it is important to acknowledge and validate suffering and abuse to lessen relational victimization of future generations, it is also important to exonerate parents and other predecessors. Exoneration is not forgiveness but understanding of parents' circumstances. It is an attempt to see another human being who also was a victim of injustice themselves and acted on their destructive entitlement in their search for justice. Of course, throughout her life and before therapy, Sonja knew the main facts of her mother's life story, but never saw her pain because her mother did not want to burden her child. She wanted, or most accurately, needed to be "strong". The therapist used the contextual therapy "seed-planting" technique through questions like "Who was there for your mom to rely on?" "Was she able to talk about her losses openly with anybody?" to facilitate a dialogue between the daughter and mother. Sonja was able to connect with her mother in a new way. Her family loyalty, mostly invisible and blocked, found a new option of expression as a family of those who, regardless of horrific circumstances, care about each other. Showing care to her elderly mom through empathy and concrete actions gave Sonja a chance to earn constructive entitlement, increased her self-worth and agency, and increased the family transgenerational "relational immune system".

Conclusion

One of the frequent consequences of multiple and prolonged sociocultural traumas such as war, oppressive political power, abrupt shifts in political and economic structures, and the hardships that follow is a decrease in basic trust. This not only impacts direct victims but can be transmitted to future generations. While the symptoms of such ongoing collective trauma are many, ranging from depression, anxiety, and low self-worth to domestic violence, substance abuse, and over- or under-protecting children, efforts to ameliorate these problems need to address the overarching assault to safety and trust—an assault that disrupts the fundamental ethical connectedness that maintains human relationships.

Ivan Boszormenyi-Nagy's contextual therapy model helps people recognize the circumstances and unfairness that befell them and their predecessors. It acknowledges the injustice—what happened to Sonja and her mother was not their "fault"; they are entitled to better. When dealing with the effects of sustained sociocultural trauma, naming the contextual nature of their suffering reduces individual blame while encouraging accountability. The approach credits Sonja's attempts to care, during her childhood and presently, and unearths and emphasizes the relational resources that Sonja and her family can activate to build trust between them and in the opportunities life holds. At the same time, beyond the domain of any one therapist, forward-thrust healing and trust building within families is potentially part of a larger parallel process of acknowledgment and restoration of community and societal bonds, with profound consequences for the future.

References

Bodrug-Lungu, V., Toma, N., & Toma, S. (2023). Sociocultural trauma among marginalized families in Moldova. In T. Glebova & C. Knudson-Martin (Eds.), *Sociocultural trauma and relational Well-being in the eastern European context (Chapter 5)*. Springer.

Boszormenyi-Nagy, I., & Krasner, B. (2014). *Between give and take: A clinical guide to contextual therapy*. Routledge. (Original work published 1986).

Boszormenyi-Nagy, I., & Sparks, G. (2013). *Invisible loyalties*. Routledge. (original work published 1984 by Brunner/mazel).

Cherepanov, E. (2021). *Understanding the transgenerational legacy of totalitarian regimes*. Routledge.

Ducommun-Nagy, C. (2018). Contextual family therapy. In J. Lebow, A. Chambers, & D. Breunlin (Eds.), *Encyclopedia of couple and family therapy* (pp. 1–8). Springer. https://doi.org/10.1007/978-3-319-15877-8_361-1

Ducommun-Nagy, C. (2021. October 13). *The resources of contextual therapy in the treatment of major mental illnesses*. International conference on contextual therapy 2021 (ICCT2021), Budapest, Hungary. https://icct2021.com/keynoters/#catherine-ducommun-nagy

Field, N. P., Moung, S., & Sochanvimean, V. (2013). Parental styles in the intergenerational transmission of trauma stemming from the Khmer rouge regime in Cambodia. *American Journal of Orthopsychiatry, 83*(4), 483–494. https://doi.org/10.1111/ajop.12057

Fonagy, P., & Allison, E. (2014). The role of mentalizing and epistemic trust in the therapeutic relationship. *Psychotherapy, 51*(3), 372–380. https://doi.org/10.1037/a0036505

Ignjatović, T. D., Hercog, N. Č., Stanković, B., & Tomanović, S. (2023). Sociocultural traumatization and resilience at the turn of the millennium: Family legacies in Serbia. In T. Glebova & C. Knudson-Martin (Eds.), *Sociocultural trauma and relational Well-being in the eastern European context (chapter 6)*. AFTA SpringerBriefs in Family Therapy,. Springer.

Knudson-Martin, C. (1992). Balancing the ledger: The applications of Nagy's theories to the study of continuity and change among generations. *Contemporary Family Therapy, 14*(3), 241–258. https://doi.org/10.1007/BF00901507

Kushner, A. (1978). One cannot choose times... (Alexander Givental, Trans.). Stihi.ru (2011). https://stihi.ru/2011/03/27/2471

Lang, A. J., & Gartstein, M. A. (2018). Intergenerational transmission of traumatization: Theoretical framework and implications for prevention. *Journal of Trauma and Dissociation, 19*(2), 162–175. https://doi.org/10.1080/15299732.2017.1329773

Lind, E. A. (2019). The study of justice in social psychology and related fields. In E. A. Lind (Ed.), *Social psychology and justice, (1st ed., pp. 1–20)*. Routledge.

Miskova, E. V. (2023). Collective trauma and retraumatization in Russia: A view from the inside. In T. Glebova & C. Knudson-Martin (Eds.), *Sociocultural trauma and relational Well-being in the eastern European context (chapter 3)*. Springer.

Papadopoulos, R. K. (2007). Refugees, trauma and adversity-activated development. *European Journal of Psychotherapy & Counseling, 9*(3), 301–312. https://doi.org/10.1080/13642530701496930

Sagi-Schwartz, A., van Ijzendoorn, M. H., & Bakermans-Kranenburg, M. J. (2008). Does intergenerational transmission of trauma skip a generation? No meta-analytic evidence for tertiary traumatization with third generation of holocaust survivors. *Attachment & Human Development, 10*(2), 105–121. https://doi.org/10.1080/14616730802113661

Sztompka, P. (2000). *Trust: A sociological theory*. Cambridge University Press.

Tarján, E., Wächter, P. P., & Wittmann, T. (2023). Historical intergenerational trauma and hope in Hungary: A contextual approach. In T. Glebova & C. Knudson-Martin (Eds.), *Sociocultural trauma and relational Well-being in the eastern European context (chapter 2)*. Springer.

Tedeschi, R. G., & Calhoun, L. G. (2004). Posttraumatic growth: Conceptual foundations and empirical evidence. *Psychological Inquiry, 15*(1), 1–18. https://doi.org/10.1207/s15327965pli1501_01

Tuck, E. (2009). Suspending damage: A letter to communities. *Harvard Educational Review, 79*(3), 409–427. https://doi.org/10.17763/haer.79.3.n0016675661t3n15

van der Meiden, J. (2019). *Where hope resides. A qualitative study of the contextual theory and therapy of Ivan Boszormenyi-Nagy and its applicability for therapy and social work.* ProefschriftMaken.

Walsh, F. (2003). Family resilience: A framework for clinical practice. *Family Process, 42*(1), 1–18. https://doi.org/10.1111/j.1545-5300.2003.00001.x

Walsh, F. (2016). Family resilience: A developmental systems framework. *European Journal of Developmental Psychology, 13*(3), 313–324. https://doi.org/10.1080/17405629.2016.1154035

Chapter 8
Clinical Work with Sociocultural Trauma

Tatiana Glebova and Carmen Knudson-Martin

As a couple and family therapist in the USA, I (Tatiana) work with many Russian-speaking immigrants, first and second generations, from the former Soviet Union, such as Russians, Ukrainians, Moldovans, and others. Their requests for professional help vary—child behavior problems, couple communication, and individual suffering, such as depression or anxiety. Along with acculturation challenges, common for many immigrants, in many cases I see the immediate and transgenerational effects of sociocultural traumas of their motherland that they "brought" with them to the new land. While this book increases attention to possible manifestations of sociocultural traumas specific to the Eastern European region, we expect it will be helpful for practitioners in many countries with histories of sociocultural traumas or admitting immigrants from those countries. Mental health professionals need to be alert to possible direct or transgenerational impacts of sociocultural traumas on individual and relational well-being; however, clinicians may not readily recognize them.

Even systemically trained clinicians use individually focused diagnoses. Consequences of prolonged and complex sociocultural traumas may appear in various forms, including anxiety, shame, and somatic complaints, to name a few; or they may resemble personality disorders, such as borderline. In relationships they may be expressed as difficulties in sustaining partnerships or problematic parent–child relationships. Seeing the sociocultural backdrop of presented clinical issues can be a challenge for clinicians both within and outside the clients' culture. Clinicians from similar cultural backgrounds may know about the historical traumas, but be

T. Glebova (✉)
Alliant International University, Sacramento, CA, USA
e-mail: tglebova@alliant.edu

C. Knudson-Martin
Emerita, Lewis & Clark College, Portland, OR, USA

T. Glebova, C. Knudson-Martin (eds.), *Sociocultural Trauma and Well-Being in Eastern European Family Therapy*, AFTA SpringerBriefs in Family Therapy,
https://doi.org/10.1007/978-3-031-29995-7_8

desensitized or numbed to them. For clinicians from a different culture, the transgenerational emergence of sociocultural trauma may not be immediately obvious or can be camouflaged as individual psychopathology or cultural values.

Eastern European cultures have been characterized as collectivistic in contrast to more individualistic Western cultures. Sociocultural traumas may produce two opposite effects on family connections—weakening or hardening. While family connections and intergenerational loyalties are an important aspect of well-being and protective factors, when they are too demanding, they can also become an obstacle to family members' individual development, especially children's. Sometimes clinicians perceive these dynamics simply as cultural and overlook their negative consequences or the sociohistorical context in which shared cultural patterns arise. Recognizing sociocultural trauma begins with third-order thinking.

Third-Order Thinking and Trauma Care

Third-order thinking (McDowell et al., 2019) broadens the lens to connect family processes and cultural patterns to sociopolitical contexts and larger systems of systems. A sociocultural trauma-informed approach applies established trauma-informed care (TIC) principles (Substance Abuse and Mental Health Services Administration, SAMHSA, 2014) within a broader contextual frame. TIC paradigm's shift from asking, "What is wrong with this person?" to "What has happened to this person?" is recast to "What has happened to this family transgenerationally and socioculturally?" Like the TIC approach, practitioners assume an individual is more likely than not to have a history of trauma, especially for clients with historical backgrounds of prolonged and drastic social changes and traumas, such as in the Eastern European region or when people live with persistent marginalization and oppression.

A sociocultural trauma-informed approach requires an explicit focus on sociocultural history, transgenerational legacies, and options for the future that transcend the dominant social system in which people were socialized. Third-order thinking starts with an assessment that links current relational symptoms within familial and societal histories and contexts. This extends to situating the therapeutic process in the social context as well. As discussed throughout this volume, one of the consequences of multiple and prolonged sociocultural trauma is a decrease of basic trust that not only impacts direct victims but can be transmitted to future generations. In addition, when historical or current social situations are characterized by societal oppression, official institutions—including mental health ones—are mistrusted. Therapists need to be prepared for low trust toward therapy and the therapist, as well as vigilance and hesitation that can be mistaken as resistance or defensiveness.

The nature of therapy entails revealing vulnerabilities, and in transgenerational work not only your own but also your family's. This can be a big challenge for those who along with several generations of their predecessors were forced by their social environment to learn that showing vulnerability is extremely dangerous. The process requires a lot of strength and courage to deal with fears, shame, and painful feelings buried inside by generations of survivors as well as dealing with visible and invisible loyalties to the family and group (see Glebova & Knudson-Martin, this volume, Chap. 7).

When Maria, 28, and Ivan, 34 (the names and some personal details are changed), California residents, asked for professional help with their relationships, they did not mention a word about "trauma." Neither reported any trauma, such as sexual assault or physical violence. Both spoke English and looked like a typical middle-class Californian White couple with common marital issues—parenting and finances. Both were perplexed and scared by the sudden and intense emotional reactions when arguing. They saw themselves as loving and caring, "good people", who wanted to have a happy family and future for their two children.

The couple felt stuck in their attempt to resolve their disagreements—any discussion of it turned to immediate emotional escalation from both sides. From a clinical diagnosis point of view, their individual reactions resembled either posttraumatic or personality disorder symptoms. But these diagnoses would be unlikely to help. On the contrary, that would confirm to them that they are "bad" and should be ashamed of themselves, especially in the context of mental health stigma widespread in their community. We could attribute these difficulties to a family system, for example, to Ivan's mom's unavailability, both physical and emotional, and make it her "problem." Alternatively, we can look at the larger systems' context, current and past, to understand the partners' predicament.

Understanding the immediate and especially long-term consequences of socially caused traumas for relationships cautions against pathologizing and attributing symptoms solely to family or individual "disorders." It does not mean that people are completely powerless or helpless against social determinants, but placing a source of trauma where it belongs is needed for justice restoration and relational healing. In fact, the importance of understanding the political context of mental health effects of massive trauma was one of the main findings of a study of newly arrived refugees from Bhutan, Burma, Ethiopia, and Somalia (Shannon et al., 2015). The researchers concluded that "acknowledging the dehumanizing nature of political oppression is healing in and of itself," especially for those who have been denied free speech (p. 453).

Silencing historical trauma, intentionally or unintentionally, at individual or societal levels may produce "postvictimization traumata" (Danieli et al., 2016) and become a barrier to healing. A "conspiracy of silence" (Danieli, 1998) has various forms and origins. In contrast, "When a [sociopolitical] past is lost in another time and in another social context, disconnected from the present, there is something profoundly validating about finally having one's experience heard" (von Sommaruga Howard, 2019, p. 237). This notion of re-storying, re-connecting, and witnessing past sociocultural traumas is relevant to relational therapy. The process begins with a proper assessment.

Assessment

Collecting a detailed historical and social background of a client, either individual or family, is especially critical for working with clients who experienced sociocultural trauma. The model of "The Impact of Sociocultural Trauma on Relational Well-Being" depicted in Fig. 1.1 (Glebova et al., this volume, Chap. 1) helps identify the complex interplay of factors across systems, with consequences that may range from resilience to severe symptoms and may contribute to or have significance for the presented problems. It is important to include the time dimension to explore both immediate and long-term impacts, as well as to be alert to generational differences in those impacts. Two well-known assessment techniques, the timeline and genogram, may serve as valuable tools.

For the timeline, the therapist should ask clients to mark meaningful events not only in a family life but also in its social environment. Clients often do not mention important sociohistorical events for a variety of reasons. The first generation may not want to talk about or even recall the past, especially if it was too traumatic. Ironically, the frequent reason for "the conspiracy of silence" around experienced traumas is an act of care, an intention to protect others, especially children. In her phenomenological study of Iraqi refugees, Gangamma (2018) found that parents struggled with simultaneously wanting to share their experience with their children and wanting to protect them from traumatization or additional hurt. At the same time, "the conspiracy of silence" is the most prevalent mechanism for the transmission of trauma. While the second and third generations may know some facts or sense a fog of secrecy in the family history, they may not see an immediate relevance of their (grand)parents' experience to their current situation. And any of them may not want to talk about those events, especially in the beginning of therapy, due to individual shame or cultural beliefs.

If a therapist shares some background like living in the same country or for some reason knows the history of the client's particular background, it can be easier to ask some open-ended but specific questions. In 2022, probably any person interested in international news around the world would know that being from Ukraine or having Ukrainian heritage signals traumatic experience, and that experience differs depending on a person's geographical location (experienced bombing/shelling or not), gender (was able to leave or not), family composition (having elderly relatives), ability, age, and SES. But probably not every therapist in the USA would be alert to possibly traumatic events in the 1990s in the former Soviet republics. Maria's parents immigrated to the USA from southern Ukraine (which was still a part of the Soviet Union) in 1991 as religious refugees just before her birth, and Ivan came much later, in 2006 as an IT professional. Clinical work with families of immigrants includes exploration of premigration, migration, and postmigration processes and stressors. Genogram and timeline assessment revealed that Maria and Ivan's current challenges were impacted by their families' histories at least two generations before immigration.

Genograms (e.g., McGoldrick et al., 2008) have been used for decades to explore and identify transgenerational processes. They visually highlight aspects of the intergenerational family system, such as cultural identity, intersectionality, or strengths. Goodman (2013) developed the Transgenerational Trauma and Resilience Genogram (TTRG) specifically to assess various forms of transgenerational trauma and guide clinical interventions that include the sociopolitical aspects of trauma and promote recovery through ecosystemic and social justice perspectives. By asking "In what ways have you, your family, or your community experienced direct, indirect, traditional, or ecosystemic stress or trauma?" (p. 392), therapists can introduce the topic with psychoeducation about those types of trauma as needed.

The source of sociocultural trauma is embedded in complex historical, social, and cultural contexts that change over time. When assessing via a timeline or genogram, a therapist needs to ask questions like "What was happening in the country or your community during that time?", "How did you or your family/parents make sense of it?", "What resources were available to you/them?", "Who did you/they turn to during the time of stress/crisis?" To make transgenerational legacies recognizable, questions like "What family rules or messages of survival or success in life, spoken and unspoken, have you received from your parents/family?" can be used.

From a contextual therapy perspective (see Glebova & Knudson-Martin, this volume, Chap. 7), identifying instances of injustice due to historical circumstances and how those led to relational injustices that may have affected family members over the generations (Ducommun-Nagy, 2018) and contribute to the current relational difficulties is important. The therapist also searches for opportunities to acknowledge social hardships of their ancestors and credit their efforts to survive, thus bringing sociocultural context and injustices into consideration with comments such as "Your grandparents went through a lot, probably it had a toll on them" or "All his life your dad worked so hard to provide for the family, but the state was taking it from him in one way or another. It's very unfair."

While a therapist may have some anticipatory ideas (and hopefully this book helps with that), clients have their own stories and views of how sociocultural forces shaped them and what might be helpful. It is also important to assess how differences, such as gender or ethnicity, interact with the social environment. For example, gender differences are internalized in social norms and behaviors. As reflected in the chapters on Russia (Miskova, this volume, Chap. 3), Moldova (Bodrug-Lungu et al., this volume, Chap. 5), and Serbia (Ignjatović, this volume, Chap. 6), gender makes a difference in how traumatic events are experienced and manifested. And people develop different coping strategies based on their strengths, abilities, and available resources.

Ivan was the only son of a single mother whose mother was a child of Russian peasants forcibly moved to Kazakhstan, then a part of the USSR, in the 1930s. The family was stripped of whatever they had—house, modest possessions, connections—and relocated to a strange faraway land where they were supposed to start from scratch somehow. His family's story was about constant physical survival, forced relocations, fear, and mistrust of the environment. Nothing was stable or secure—resources, support, or connections with other people. Ivan's most vivid and painful memories were about his school years in the middle of 1990s with its economic crisis after the collapse of the Soviet Union. His mom wasn't receiving even the minimal salary that she had before. She tried to find ways to provide for her son and herself, moved several times in search of work, and rarely was home.

Ivan focused on his studies, was able to attend and graduate from college due to his math abilities, and left the country as soon as he was able. His primary motivation was to escape poverty and never remember it. His motto "You can rely only on yourself; everyone's for themselves" was even beneficial in his adjustment to US professional norms and success. Other beliefs such as "it's better not to speak up" and "I don't deserve anything" prevented him from asking for a raise or saying "no" to extra work given to him, since he was very responsible and hardworking. So, while he wanted his children to have a life different from his childhood, he, like his mom and grandma, was rarely around them, being mostly preoccupied with his work, and when they or his wife complained about it, Ivan's response would be "What's wrong with you? You have everything." Ivan felt stressed out, anxious, but when anybody asked "How are you?" his typical reply "I'm fine, not complaining" was also a perfect fit for American culture.

Maria also grew up in poverty in more or less the same time period. She was the oldest daughter of five of parents whose evangelical Christian community experienced various forms of persecution and discrimination in the former Soviet Union. They left the USSR for religious freedom when changes in both Soviet emigration and US refugee policies (1988) made it possible. They carried very few physical possessions but heavy mental "baggage" with them—mistrust toward governments and "others," thinking that only family and church community could be trusted. Maria's role was to help with younger siblings and around the house. She learned how to "read minds" of her younger siblings and mom. Maria's family history included starvation during the mass famine of Holodomor in Ukraine (great-grandparents), occupation by the Nazis and fighting during World War II, and rebuilding their lives after the war. Focus on providing food and saving their resources were the family's survival strategy. Loyalty to one's family, close connection, and self-sacrifice for others were main familial values. Children were expected to follow very strict rules and have limited freedom beyond the family for the sake of their own safety, since the world outside of home was dangerous.

For several generations, Maria and Ivan's families experienced multiple and severe sociocultural traumas and developed relevant survival strategies. Beliefs like "Nobody can be trusted" and "The future is unpredictable" came from people's life experiences. Messages like "You are nothing/not important," "speaking up for yourself (or just speaking) is dangerous" were actively propagated by the society, from slogans to schooling. This collective survival history led to a "heroic and stoic" identity—we can survive anything, endless patience is a virtue; strength is in silence; poor people are noble; caring about yourself is shameful; sacrifice for others is the biggest honor.

All those messages and learned responses were at work when the partners tried to discuss their issues or when "little things" during everyday life triggered emotional memories. The escalations were fast and left both deeply hurt, confused, and ashamed. Maria would cry, Ivan would apologize, and both would try to avoid any "conflict" till the next trigger and emotional outburst. They started to distance themselves from each other, feeling diminished and distrustful of each other or even themselves. As many couples seeking therapy, they wanted to resolve their communication problems. It took some time before they started to share their families' stories; in the beginning (when we did a basic genogram), they did not want to talk much about it.

It became clear that interactions of past social and familial messages were making it difficult for Maria and Ivan to create a secure and trustworthy connection with each other. Speaking up for yourself, expressing your needs and emotions, or asking for help was prohibited. During peaceful periods both, but especially Maria, were trying to anticipate the partner's needs and desires and expected the same from the partner. When they fell in love, they hoped that the other would be a source of ideal endless love that would compensate for the non-received care of their childhoods. During conflicts, this focus channeled into blaming the other. Their destructive entitlements from the past made them feel justified in focusing on their own pain without considering the partner's—"You don't care about me, so I don't care about you." Maria struggled with split loyalty between her tightly connected family of origin and her husband, while Ivan's loyalty to his family legacy was mostly invisible.

Restoring Connectedness and Building Trust

This volume's chapters show not only a variability of societal contexts and clinical issues that stem from sociocultural trauma but also a variability of therapeutic approaches to address them. Individual and family attachment-based models, contextual therapy, narrative, internal family systems, body-focused work, group therapy, and psychodrama are illustrated by authors in this book. There is no one perfect model, and interventions may focus on different systemic levels. All focus on alleviating the assaults to social bonds and identities perpetuated by war, oppression, and other forms of collective fear.

Processing and healing from sociocultural traumas happen within social and state structures with their current political and ideological dynamics. At the state level, some historical events are acknowledged and often amplified, while others are concealed. In societies or communities where social trauma is heavily silenced or there are no words for its expression, less verbal approaches can be more acceptable. Symbolic and artistic modes provide effective means of processing past traumas at both individual and social levels. Existence or creation of memorials or museums dedicated to traumatic social pasts validates survivors' experiences and create a public space of acknowledgment and remembrance for future generations.

The relevance of social processing for individual and familial healing was detailed in Chap. 2 on Hungary (Tarján et al., this volume). Various forms of collective work, such as group therapy or performing arts like backstage theater, are also pertinent to the nature of sociocultural trauma as a collective experience and can provide some social context and connections for rectifying the impact of sociocultural trauma. Available types of healing, traditional or institutionalized ones, depend on the culture and current social situation. However, they all highlight a critical principle—restoring trustworthy connections with themselves, with family and community members as well as with therapists, as a resource for overcoming destructive relational consequences of sociocultural trauma.

Clinical Guiding Principles

Trauma-Informed Care emphasizes safety, collaboration, compassion, strength-focus, and prevention of retraumatization (SAMHSA, 2014). A sociocultural trauma-informed approach incorporates these within a third-order lens that emphasizes relational justice guided by the following clinical principles.

Trustworthiness

Regardless of a particular modality, clinical work with people who experienced sociocultural trauma places paramount importance on establishing trusting relationships and instilling hope for the future. In contextual therapy, this principle is explicit as a therapy goal and foundation (Boszormenyi-Nagy & Krasner, 1986/2014). With clients whose family history for decades was teaching them "don't trust," this can be easier said than done. As simple as it may sound, the first step is a detailed discussion of what to expect from counseling or therapy, and the role you play as a therapist. It is important to ask about previous experience of counseling. Whether they had therapy before or not, the topic of trust needs to be brought up; it is especially critical for those seeking professional help for the first time. I (Tatiana) sometimes spend a large portion of the first session discussing how clients feel about sharing their personal issues and how their family or friends may see it. I normalize clients' possible hesitancy to open up by saying, "For many people it is really difficult, especially with a complete stranger." Discussion of the confidentiality policy and its exceptions requires detailed attention. Those discussions set a foundation for safety and collaboration in therapy.

Like socioculturally attuned family therapy (McDowell et al., 2023), the sociocultural trauma-informed approach is transtheoretical; various models and methods such as attachment, narrative, solution-focused, cognitive-behavioral, internal family systems, and others can be used under the umbrella of relational justice. While linking presented issues to the larger social and historical context, it is important to address symptoms directly connected to clients' presented issues and desired goals and to be attuned to their language and worldview. Some immediate and specific symptom relief can strengthen the therapist's trustworthiness and give hope for change.

For example, Maria and Ivan had emotionally volatile and heated arguments. One of the short-term treatment goals was to decrease emotional reactivity by giving them some tools to prevent escalations and regulate their own emotions. As the clients noted, sessions themselves provided them with a new experience of calmer and more meaningful dialogues. Also, psychoeducation regarding emotions and ways to identify them (bodily sensations, thoughts, and behaviors) and techniques to regulate them were provided (similar to work with PTSD symptoms, for example, developed by Cloitre and colleagues and applied to clinical work with refugees (Tissue et al., 2022)). Each small improvement and change increases clients' sense of agency and control, as well as trust in self and significant others, that were diminished generationally.

Prevention of Retraumatization

Sociocultural trauma-informed work entails alertness in anticipating and avoiding practices that are likely to retraumatize people who already have histories of trauma. One retraumatization risk is a "pathologizing" and "labeling" stance. It is essential that therapists avoid a judgmental and shame-inducing attitude, including characterizing clients as resistant. Some clients may not want to be labeled depressed or anxious because they have a family legacy of being strong and overcoming hardships. Sometimes even an expression of any "negative" feelings such as sadness or hopelessness is prohibited in families of survivors whose positive attitudes helped them to overcome traumas.

Strength-Based

Amidst the violence of war and man-made destruction, many people find ways to help each other and express their care through actions. My friends in Ukraine tell me they hardly knew some of their neighbors before the war, but since it began neighbors help each other in many ways. It happens at many levels, including internationally; other countries and their people open their homes to refugees and organize other ways to support them. Mental health professionals have established systems to provide immediate psychological support to those who need it in and outside Ukraine. Children in Ukraine, the future generation, not only suffer various losses but show adults and sometimes surprise them with their expressions of concern and care about others. One woman shared a story on social media that when she was sitting with others in the shelling shelter she heard a boy, around 5 years of age, asking how much he can drink from the water bottle, so there would be enough left for others. There are many similar stories around the world. They are "witness to humanity" not only of possible horrors, but also of existing hope and human concern for fairness and care.

From the very beginning, the therapist's task is active listening for strengths and acts of care, not only of clients in the room but their families as well. For example, with Maria and Ivan it was critical to acknowledge their courage to ask for help that showed that they care about each other. During the genogram and family history conversation both Maria's and Ivan's families were discussed from a strength-based perspective.

Exploration of Family Legacy

In working with transgenerational trauma, exploring family legacies can be especially helpful. This can be done throughout the therapy, when relevant, by asking questions like "How is your thought/emotion/action related to your family history?" Then it is important to connect it with the present—"How is your situation different now?" and "What part of your family legacy is helpful now and what belongs to the past?" This work can be done in a special session if clients see it as important, using various visual or symbolic techniques, depending on clients' preferences, such as "sorting out family baggage or chest"—"What is given to me?", "What is there?", "What do you want to keep?", "How can it be helpful for you now?", "What do I want to leave for posterity/children?"

Agency and Accountability

Placing a cause of destructive (in the current context) behaviors in the realm of the broader social system may create a tension between "agency" and "helplessness." At the extreme points, people (including therapists and clients) may have a tendency to either see behaviors as fully historically determined or fully under control of people (blaming others, including family members, or feeling extremely guilty themselves). Prolonged sociocultural disruptions are mostly beyond people's control. In addition, totalitarian regimes intentionally control the public and private lives of their citizens to destroy their agency and willpower. Survival messages like "Nothing is under our control" can be empathically challenged by discussing what actually is under at least some control, for instance, a way of relating to your partner or children.

When working with Maria and Ivan on their communication, we examined their relational expectations in the context of family history. Their expectations that the other would serve as a source of unconditional love and attention stemmed from under-given care in their childhoods and were not fair to their partner. Collaboratively we sorted out what they can fairly give and receive from each other. Empowering clients to be accountable for their actions by expressing their own needs while hearing the other side gives them a sense of agency and control. This gradually leads to strengthening their relational resource—trust built on trustworthy actions of mutual fair relating.

Concern for the Future Generations

Transgenerational trauma requires attention not only to the past and the present but intentional therapeutic work to minimize its transmission to future generations. Maria and Ivan had two children. Even though their main presented issues were not directly about the kids, a therapist concerned about the future, such as a contextual therapist (see Glebova & Knudson-Martin, this volume, Chap. 7), will bring it up. This imperative is supported by research. In clinical recommendations based on the critical review of studies on traumatized parents with symptoms of posttraumatic stress disorder, the parent–child interaction, and the impact on their nonexposed child, Van Ee et al. (2016) concluded that "Clinicians of traumatized parents have the responsibility to inquire about the client's parenting and their child" (p. 198). Maria and Ivan were responsive to the therapist's questions, such as "What do your children do when they see you upset or arguing?", and expressed their concern about an impact on children that was acknowledged and supported by the therapist. We talked about what they want for their children and what they as parents can do now to support their children's future. The parents were able to see how some of their expectations, such as that the children would always be nice and well-behaved, were unrealistic and unfair.

Investment in the future does not give immediate results. It takes time to grow. It is why a contextual approach to sociocultural trauma includes seed planting and moratorium principles (Boszormenyi-Nagy & Krasner, 1986/2014). Through planting the seed of fairer relating, the therapist opens family's relational resources, but it is family members whose energy will create trust and health. A moratorium takes into consideration clients' readiness and timing and gives them a choice when and how to implement their accountability. This approach of respecting clients' decision-making process is in strong accordance with TIC. Therapists need to be prepared for an ongoing nonlinear process that may not have a full "resolution" by the end of formal treatment.

Self-of-Therapist

Being a caring and relationally insightful person is not enough. Empathy and perspective-taking should go beyond clients' emotional or living experience and include apprehension of clients' perceptions of therapists and therapy within a larger social context (McDowell et al., 2023). They need to be aware of their own culture as a worldview, expectations of others and reactions to different frames of living, and keep learning about themselves. For example, a therapist who deeply and strongly shares the US dominant culture's belief that the future is under our control (through self-determination, goal setting, and hard work) might negatively react to Maria and Ivan's shared belief that the world is unpredictable and anything, mostly meaning something harmful, can happen at any moment. This belief became reinforced during sudden sociocultural traumas, such as the Covid-19 pandemic and the war in Ukraine.

It can be tricky, for both therapists and clients, to keep a balance between understanding the long-lasting impacts of social traumas and giving clients agency and control over defining what their challenge is. Various forms of consultations, formal or peer, are needed. Knowing your own transgenerational and personal trauma history and signs of possible retraumatization or secondary traumatization, as well as the impact of the therapist's own sociocultural context on worldviews and what is taken for granted as normal, is integral to equitable and competent socioculturally attuned practice (McDowell et al., 2023).

Conclusion

The principles for sociocultural trauma-informed practice offered here call on therapists to regularly expand the lens through which they see, interpret, and respond to client symptoms. Failing to recognize the sociopolitical contexts of clients' troubles and habitual ways of relating perpetuates the trauma. While interventions that mitigate some of the immediate symptoms are helpful and important, healing from the effects of sociocultural trauma does not happen quickly and involves helping clients envision a new path forward for themselves and those who follow. Acknowledgment of the contextual nature of the shared trauma is validating and important. It is also important to guard against simplification and overgeneralization by attuning to each person's unique experience within the collective trauma. As trust builds, new connections are supported and mutually caring relationships based on accountability and fairness are possible.

References

Bodrug-Lungu, V., Toma, N., & Toma, S. (2023). Sociocultural trauma among marginalized families in Moldova. In T. Glebova & C. Knudson-Martin (Eds.), *Sociocultural trauma and relational Well-being in the eastern European context (Chapter 5)*. Springer.

Boszormenyi-Nagy, I., & Krasner, B. (2014). *Between give and take: A clinical guide to contextual therapy*. Routledge. (Original work published 1986).

Danieli, Y. (1998). Introduction: History and conceptual foundations. In Y. Danieli (Ed.), *International handbook of multigenerational legacies of trauma* (pp. 1–20). Plenum.

Danieli, Y., Norris, F. H., & Engdahl, B. (2016). Multigenerational legacies of trauma: Modeling the what and how of transmission. *American Journal of Orthopsychiatry, 86*(6), 639–651. https://doi.org/10.1037/ort0000145

Ducommun-Nagy, C. (2018). Contextual family therapy. In J. Lebow, A. Chambers, & D. Breunlin (Eds.), *Encyclopedia of couple and family therapy* (pp. 1–8). Springer. https://doi.org/10.1007/978-3-319-15877-8_361-1
Gangamma, R. (2018). A phenomenological study of family experiences of resettled Iraqi refugees. *Journal of Marital and Family Therapy, 44*(2), 323–335. https://doi.org/10.1111/jmft.12251
Glebova, K.-M., & Glebov, K. (2023). Introduction: Sociocultural trauma and relational Well-being in the Eastern European context. In T. Glebova & C. Knudson-Martin (Eds.), *Sociocultural trauma and relational Well-being in the Eastern European context (chapter 1)*. Springer.
Glebova, T., & Knudson-Martin, C. (2023). Sociocultural trauma and intergenerational relational ethics. In T. Glebova & C. Knudson-Martin (Eds.), *Sociocultural trauma and relational Well-being in the Eastern European context (chapter 7)*. Springer.
Goodman, R. D. (2013). The transgenerational trauma and resilience genogram. *Counseling Psychology Quarterly, 26*(3–4), 386–405. https://doi.org/10.1080/09515070.2013.820172
Ignjatović, T.d., Hercog, N. Č., Stanković, B., & Tomanović, S. (2023). Sociocultural traumatization and resilience at the turn of the millennium: Family legacies in Serbia. In T. Glebova & C. Knudson-Martin (Eds.), *Sociocultural trauma and relational Well-being in the eastern European context (chapter 6)*. Springer.
McDowell, T., Knudson-Martin, C., & Bermudez, M. (2019). Toward third thinking in family therapy: Addressing social justice across family therapy practice. *Family Process, 58*, 9–22. https://doi.org/10.1111/famp.12383
McDowell, T., Knudson-Martin, C., & Bermudez, M. (2023). *Socioculturally attuned family therapy: Toward equitable theory and practice* (2nd ed.). Routledge.
McGoldrick, M., Gerson, R., & Petry, S. (2008). *Genograms: Assessment and intervention* (3rd ed.). Norton.
Shannon, P. J., Wieling, E., McCleary, J. S., & Becher, E. (2015). Exploring the mental health effects of political trauma with newly arrived refugees. *Qualitative Health Research, 25*(4), 443–457. https://doi.org/10.1177/1049732314549475
Substance Abuse and Mental Health Services Administration. (2014). *Trauma-informed care in behavioral health services*. Treatment Improvement Protocol (TIP) Series 57. HHS PublicationNo. (SMA) 13–4801. Substance Abuse and Mental Health Services Administration.
Tarján, E., Wächter, P. P., & Wittmann, T. (2023). Historical intergenerational trauma and hope in Hungary: A contextual approach. In T. Glebova & C. Knudson-Martin (Eds.), *Sociocultural trauma and relational Well-being in the Eastern European context (chapter 2)*. Springer.
Tissue, A., Specker, P., Hoffman, J., Uppal, S., Cloitre, M., Neuner, F., & Nickerson, A. (2022). Skills training in affective and interpersonal regulation for refugees integrated with narrative exposure therapy: A case study on the treatment of PTSD and emotion dysregulation for refugees and asylum-seekers. *Clinical Case Studies*, 1–21. https://doi.org/10.1177/15346501221133315
van Ee, E., Kleber, R. J., & Jongmans, M. J. (2016). Relational patterns between caregivers with PTSD and their nonexposed children: A review. *Trauma, Violence, & Abuse, 17*(2), 186–203. https://doi.org/10.1177/1524838015584355
von Sommaruga Howard, T. (2019). Sociopolitical trauma: Forgetting, remembering, and group analysis. *Transactional Analysis Journal, 49*(4), 233–247. https://doi.org/10.1080/03621537.2019.1649846

Appendix

See Maps A.1, A.2, A.3 and A.4 below:

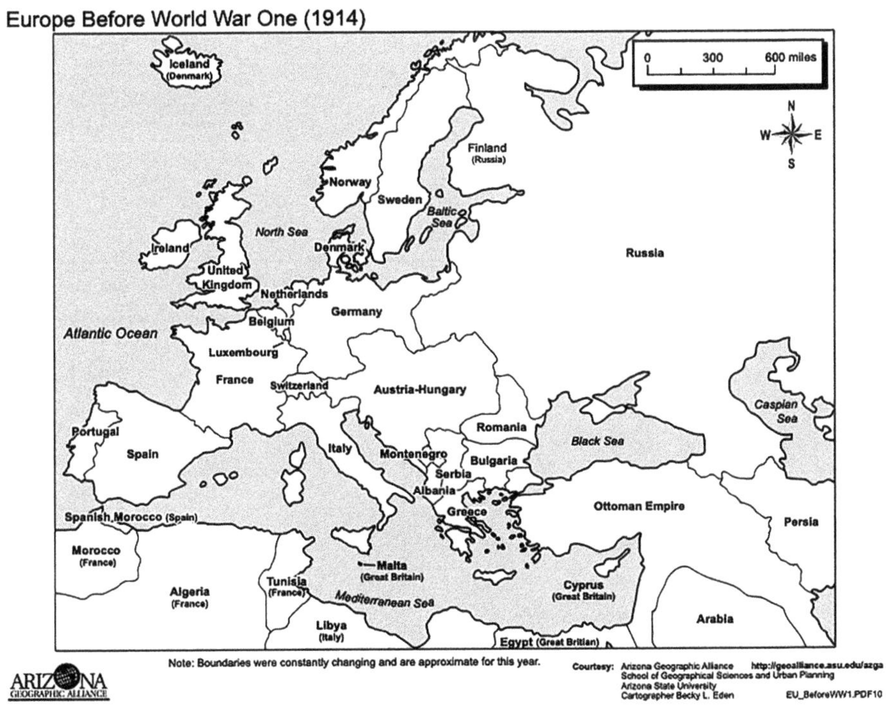

Map A.1 Map of Europe before World War I (1914)

T. Glebova, C. Knudson-Martin (eds.), *Sociocultural Trauma and Well-Being in Eastern European Family Therapy*, AFTA SpringerBriefs in Family Therapy,
https://doi.org/10.1007/978-3-031-29995-7

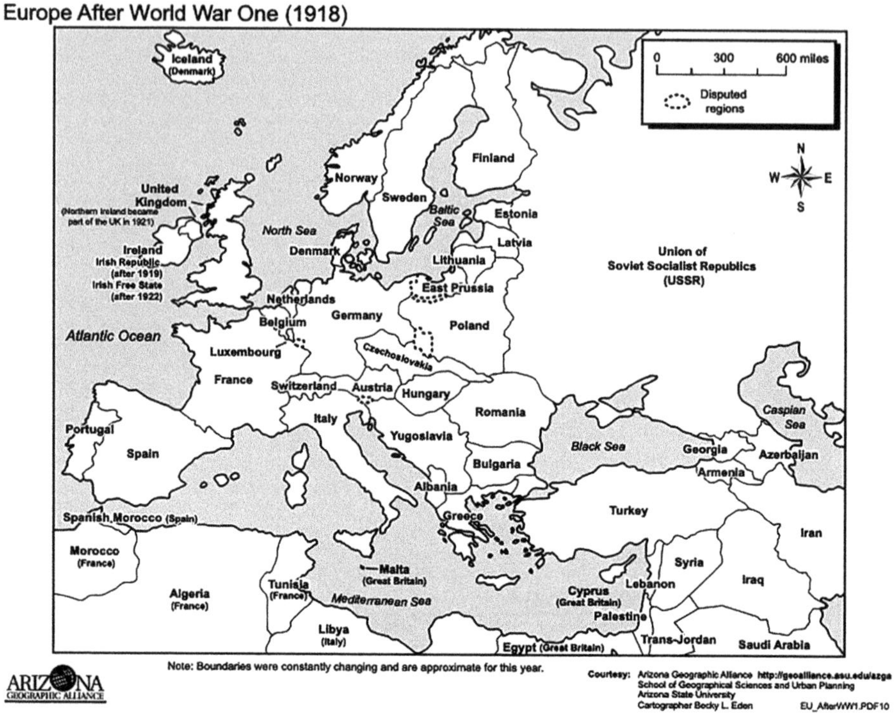

Map A.2 Europe after World War I (1918)

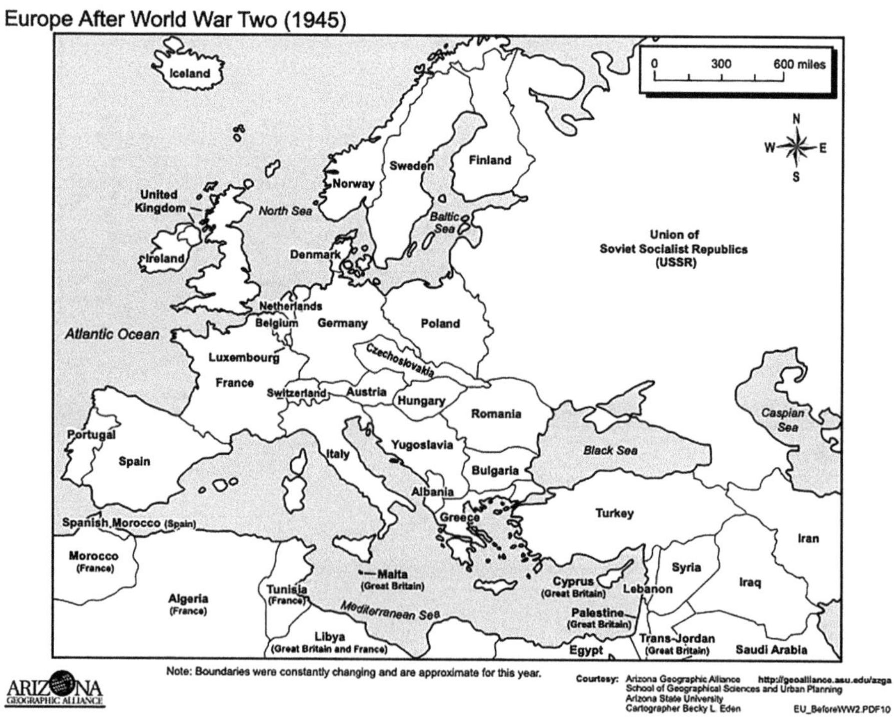

Map A.3 Europe after World War II (1945)

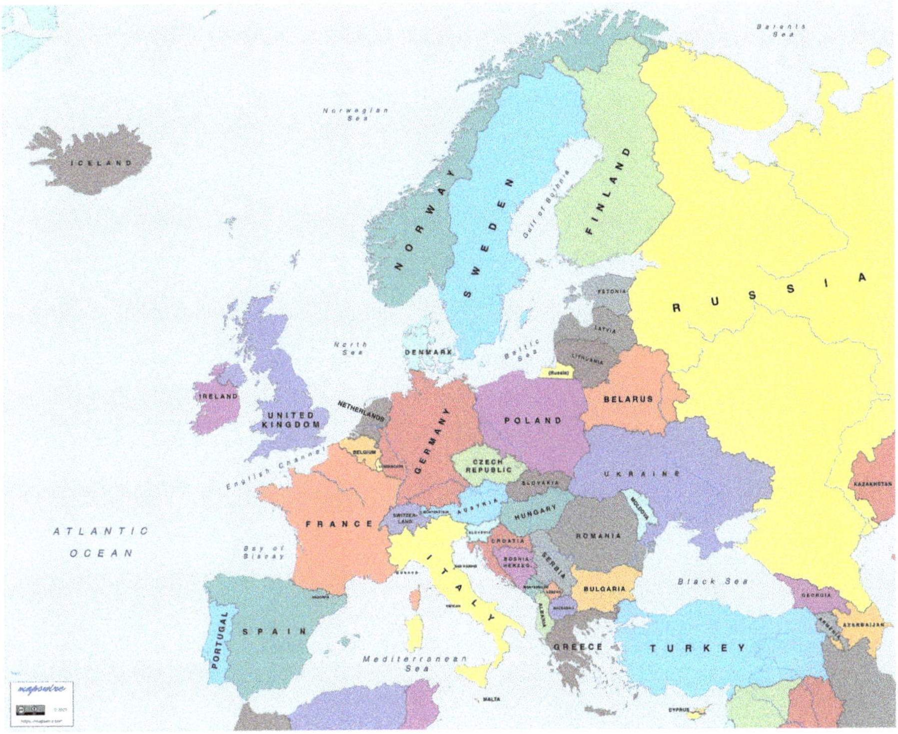

Map A.4 Europe, Current (2022)

Index

T. Glebova, C. Knudson-Martin (eds.), *Sociocultural Trauma and Well-Being in Eastern European Family Therapy*, AFTA SpringerBriefs in Family Therapy, https://doi.org/10.1007/978-3-031-29995-7

GPSR Compliance
The European Union's (EU) General Product Safety Regulation (GPSR) is a set of rules that requires consumer products to be safe and our obligations to ensure this.

If you have any concerns about our products, you can contact us on

ProductSafety@springernature.com

In case Publisher is established outside the EU, the EU authorized representative is:

Springer Nature Customer Service Center GmbH
Europaplatz 3
69115 Heidelberg, Germany

www.ingramcontent.com/pod-product-compliance
Ingram Content Group UK Ltd.
Pitfield, Milton Keynes, MK11 3LW, UK
UKHW020704041026
15590UKWH00001B/461

* 9 7 8 3 0 3 1 2 9 9 9 4 0 *